You Are Bigger
Than the Pain

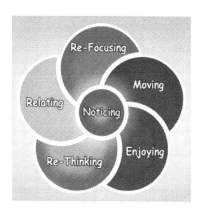

Six Comfort Strategies for
People in Chronic Pain

Daniel Lev, Ph.D.

Comfort Skills Press – Kailua, Hawaii
©2018

Lev, Daniel, 1953 –

Margaret Walkover, Chief Editor
Beth Lynne, Interior Layout & Design
Publish and Promote, InDesign Layout
Laura LaRoche, Cover Design
Creative 7 Designs, Front Cover Graphics

Printed and bound in the USA
ISBN 978-0-692-94578-0 (Paperback)
ISBN 978-0-692-08576-9 (eBook)

Note to reader: The information included in this book is accurate and complete according to the best of the author's knowledge. However, all the information is presented without guarantee on the part of the author or publisher, who also disclaim any liability in connection with the use of this information.

Contents

Preface

I met Daniel about 5 years ago in the context of mutual studies related to the management of pain. We are each mature professionals who have dedicated decades of our careers seeking to better understand available options to help others overcome painful physiological conditions. My own background in nursing -- including working with individuals in the last stages of life, and in counseling individuals with chronic conditions has given me in-depth exposure to the magnitude of need. My own strong background in clinical hypnosis has taught me that intense suffering can be reversed and individuals can learn to recapture lost hope with their own internal resiliency. It is a matter of learning. Daniel Lev and I found common ground in our optimism and our ideas that the body and mind hold within untapped resources that can be redirected to serve this urgent need.

It is with great pleasure that I now read the completed volume *You are Bigger than the Pain*. Having immersed myself in literature about pain management for over half a century I can attest that Lev's work provides a comprehensive approach coming in from a rarely explored direction. Instead of avoiding pain, Lev advocates active pursuit of comfort. This important work provides an opportunity for individuals to redirect their own present and future to a comfortable sense of normalcy.

Daniel Lev's book is as informative as it is captivating. This volume focuses on recognition of one's own capacity to create and maintain comfort even when confronted by trying circumstances. In so doing, Lev also addresses one of the great contributors to the experience of pain -- the sense of helplessness related to the way that pain draws energy, resources and possibility for change *away* from the sufferer.

In contrast to more traditional approaches to working with pain -- which generally aspire to management through control or avoidance of painful physical sensations -- Lev's approach emphasizes the development of a hypnotic mindset. His unique work begins with a foundation of rational thinking, understanding and behavioral adjustments. From this solid beginning, the creative redirection continues to expand using evidence-based stories, explanations, and exercises. The powerful potential of suggestion, working with expectations, and of self-monitored states of conscious awareness provide fertile opportunity for change. Conscious alterations of one's focus of attention can evolve into a shift in unconscious perspective wherein comfort itself becomes the focal point.

You are Bigger than the Pain acknowledges that pain can be powerful, frightening, and insidious and can even take over one's life with a self-reinforcing process that increases sensitivity instead of reducing it. Pain does that, and thus we have huge populations of individuals whose lives are compromised. Frequently, the individual then seeks relief through control (medications and procedures), through avoidance, denial or distraction. Some clinicians advocate acceptance as another approach to this problem; however, in Lev's experience, most clients shy away from this option, choosing to actively to alter their situation. All of these are strategies that continue with discomfort in the lead. Lev proposes to turn this around, and put comfort in the leading role.

Pain is complex in its expression; individuals are complex in their responses. Lev's considerable efforts to be comprehensive with his studies involved years in the making. His clinical experiences in therapeutic pain management settings led him to a seemingly inexhaustible conundrum -- the individuality of the expression of pain, coupled with personalized attempts to mitigate the sensations. This work reflects Lev's in-depth examination of the world of those who have been trapped in the redundancy of a pain experience. What Lev found was that despite all of the observations, information and resources, and individual attempts at adaptation -- a large segment of the population in need were left underserved by available resources. Thus the inspiration for Lev to transcribe his wisdom into a readable, manageable guide that can reach out to people in need, both near and far.

You are Bigger than the Pain provides an innovative guide for release from the loop of discomfort, distress and confinement. The strength of this work is also its weakness. Lev sought to make it as comprehensive as possible. This noble goal led to an expansive unwieldy treatise. Driven by his own commitment, he sought to refine the massive information into a meaningful collection of concepts -- the overriding and most central core concept being emphasis on comfort.

Lev's thesis is that through working with individual capacity to enhance one's own comfort, there is a natural progression of pain reduction. As one's focus of attention is consciously altered, the internal and unconscious perspective of misery shifts – and as this happens, pain sensitivity in the nervous system calms down, leading to increased comfort. The pain settles into a context more fitting to the overall life experience. In other words, acceptance of the presence of pain can be concurrent with a redirection of attention into an active pursuit of comfort. This action on the part of the sufferer stimulates a neuro-plastic cascade that leads to a more adaptive lifestyle as well as enhancement of quality of life. That positive redirection becomes a new directive for the life experience providing a fulfilling cycle of displacement of the maladaptive spiral. Little by little, the individuals become empowered in their own capacity to focus where they choose, and the disempowered pain recedes.

Pain may continue to have a presence within one's life, but learning to work around such an intruder can substantially alter the qualitative life experience. Yet rallying the energy for re-direction can be challenging in its own way. The enhancement of comfort involves an entire experiential deviation; it involves habitual responses, emotions, daily schedules, social response and self-reflection. It requires time, self-exploration, awareness of the signals the body produces and a learned ability to assess the signals. It involves a contemplation of what comfort feels like, a search for meaningful experiences to draw from, and an ongoing supply of hope for a harmonious life experience. It involves learning to work with one's own conscious and unconscious internal resources in a meaningful and deliberate way.

This book offers a tutorial for how to develop needed skills. The concepts are available for individuals who haphazardly open the book to scan the contents, for those who just want a quick fix, and for those who are willing to make a commitment of dedicated effort to redirect their lives. The book partitions extensive reading separately from the boot-camp intensive; it is arranged in a style to facilitate finding a path that works for the reader regardless of their readiness to make a commitment. The formatting into sections is at once directive and permissive. It invites the reader to find one's own direction. This choice-making helps position the reader on a path to stabilize life areas that may need serious re-direction. Even the floral logo reminds participants of different facets of the journey by subtly suggesting directions available to address any present discomfort.

This work brings together the wisdom Lev gleaned from the most reliable sources -- those in pain. It combines his passion for helping others with the considerable knowledge amassed and now organized into meaningful lessons that guide participants through the process of change. Daniel Lev's work is a masterful collection of skills woven together with innovative thinking and a permissive perspective that opens a door to invite change.

Roxanna Erickson-Klein RN, LPC, PhD.
Dallas Texas

Foreword

You Are Bigger Than the Pain comes at an opportune time, when opioid addiction has become a problem of epidemic proportions. Some of this is due to increased marketing of analgesic medication combined with the inability of stressed medical personnel to spend time with their patients and offer alternatives. Surely, though, the rise in the use of opioids also reflects a rise in the prevalence of chronic pain. Pain is always both physical and psychological; these days at least some of the pain is also existential. A good deal of the misery comes as a result of our materialist, consumerist times. When people are treated as customers and pain relief is treated as a commodity, both patients and doctors lose patience: rapid gratification becomes a substitute for caring for ourselves and for others.

While there is nothing inherently wrong in using analgesics appropriately for pain relief, medications alone are never a solution for life's ills. Ingesting anodynes – pain killing drugs - whether they be opioids or the latest fad for a quick fix - reflects a loss of faith in ourselves and others. Our relationships start being judged only by their results - does it make me feel good? - and we forget that pain is not the same as suffering. Ultimately we must find agency and make sense of our experience not so much in the pleasant or unpleasant contents of the events we encounter, but in how we face the fluctuations of our lives and mold them to meaning.

Daniel Lev reminds everyone that even when our lives are marked by hurt and even anguish, these are never the whole story. Lev's message is clear - comfort is possible; that the warmth of intimacy trumps the cold hurt of isolation; that each person is an unfolding story, a living being rather than a number on a medical chart. This comfort approach adds immeasurably to the usual strategies of medical treatments, personal endurance and purely rational approaches which enjoin us to talk back to our pain. These can all be useful. But Dr. Lev in this book expands our repertoire by appealing not just to reason, but also to our imagination, our hearts and spirits. These offer power and comfort which, even when we have forgotten them in our sleep of pain, are always within reach just like the pillow we grope for in the dark of night.

By reminding us that we our bigger than our pain, Dr. Lev offers us an opportunity to wake up to our full potential even in the midst of our difficulties. His mixture of empathy, practical advice and down-to-earth humor make *You Are Bigger Than the Pain* an invaluable resource for anyone who needs to deal with pain, and for the people who care for them. Reading this book and putting it into practice will enable you to get moving and change your relationship to pain, to re-focus and re-think your troubles. Most important, it will help you appreciate your life. Enjoy!

Robert Rosenbaum, PhD
Author of "Zen and the Art of Psychotherapy," and
"Walking the Way: 81 Zen Encounters with the Tao Te Ching"

People-in-Pain Speak Out about Comfort Skills

Nancy S:

Dr Lev's program (and his book) should be used by all those dealing with chronic illness. Working with him has changed my life in more ways than I can count including: avoiding flares by noticing triggers, identifying and planning strategies to deal with the people that cause stress and anxiety in my life, and planning positive activities to look forward to on my good days. Using his skills and guidance has allowed me to significantly reduce my pain and stress, as well as teaching me a better way to deal with all of the areas of my life that are impacted by my chronic illnesses. I just wish I'd had his help and tools over 20-year ago!

Kathleen S:

If you are lucky enough in your life to meet a professional in charge of making you feel better, who actually sees you, really sees you for who and what you are, then I believe you would have met someone like Dr Lev. I remember the first day that he walked into a support group I attended called 'The Comfort Circle.' I thought

> *"Who is this guy? Are you kidding me?! - He came with Buddhist meditation beads, a yarmulke, a little stomach, in casual cloths. Am I in the wrong place?"*

Well, it turned out that I was in the right place. This man taught me so much about myself, about my pain. Self hypnosis (before, no one could hypnotize me), being one of the most valuable tools. Dr Lev taught us to understand our pain conditions. For me it means a cooperative life with my pain, learning to live a normal ("New Normal") life realizing that I would be living with it for a long time so I might as well befriend it. Together we found classes, doctors, and procedures to further assist in my strengthening my spine.

I never left an appointment, or a Comfort Circle without feeling better, experiencing less pain, and most importantly, always laughing. I will never be pain free, however now I am not totally controlled by it.

Susan T:

I have been in Dr. Lev's Comfort Skills Class for a year now and I must say he has literally provided me with the knowledge, tools, ability and the strength to enhance my mind, body and soul to look outside the box and learn a new way of life to deal with chronic pain through Hypnosis and Meditation. Before I met this amazing man I was suffering tremendously, taking a lot of pain, inflammation, nerve, and sleeping medications. Now, I am only on nerve pills and occasional one pain pill. The Meditation and Hypnosis techniques he teaches provided me with the relaxation and mind control that helps me control a lot of my own pain. Dr. Lev provides not only the techniques, but a relationship with you to guide you through your personal understanding of your mind to body.

There are many hypnosis techniques that he has taught me but my favorite is the "Eye Lid Drop." It is the easiest way for me to focus on one spot and allow my eyes to let my mind relax. As my eyes get tired and my body and mind catch up the eye lids get tired of staying open and they get dry and start to close. I cannot keep them open and I drift off. Simple as that! I also use his audio recordings - his voice is amazing, so soothing, calming and peaceful!

Dr. Lev is a miracle and his craft has been a gift to me as well as to all who I have had the honor of sharing his classes with. I love going to his class just to relax with my class mates and share our stories and experiences together! I can't speak for them, but I LOVE knowing that Tuesday is coming and I have that class to go to for comfort.

Sharon W:

I think the Comfort Skills should be called survival skills. This is because they help me get through flares and fearful thoughts. My favorite is hypnosis although I use the breathing technique for emergencies. When you find your favorite techniques practice them regularly so they become automatic when needed. I like to use the hypnosis recording as a timer. This can help in two ways. At night when the pain is sharpest for me, I play the first recording. If the pain hasn't eased up I play the second recording. After that I've either started to fall asleep or the pain level has dropped. It also works for naps. The more I practice it the better it works for pain reduction.

Carolyn A:

For far too many years I have suffered with chronic pain due to degenerated spinal discs and sciatica. My quality of life was greatly diminished and the worst part was feeling that my doctors didn't really believe me...so many times I was dismissed, diminished, or told it was all in my head. Finally I found a doctor who sent me to the Chronic Pain Program where I met Dr. Daniel Lev. The first day of the program I heard the words I needed: "We know your pain is real, we're going to help you." Relief and validation flooded through me. I knew that this was the program which would help me find my "new normal."

The program combined pain management, physical therapy, mental therapy, meditation and reassurance. I found that with the multiple tools I'd learned, I could be in charge! I came up with strategies to manage even the bad days; such as my comfort box. In it I placed anything relaxing or pleasurable, like candles, books, music, journal, blanket, etc. Chronic pain does have to control your life! Learn the tools you need to manage it and Be Blessed!

Appreciations

First, I reserve my greatest appreciation for the brave souls I have met along this journey who struggle with pain and its related problems every day. I learned my deepest lessons from them, their stories and inspiration are included on every page, and they are the true authors of this book.

It took me twelve years to finish this book. I could not have brought it to completion without the inspiration and support of a number of amazing individuals. First, I want to thank, from the bottom of my heart, my buddy Hal Aronson for encouraging me to do the "Big Push" and write the whole book in 6-days (paralleling G-d). Although those days have stretched into years, I appreciate his advice to stop hunting for a publisher and just "write the book."

I'm very appreciative of Dr. Kevin Cheng, pharmacist Janny Lee, psychologist Pat Dwyer and others at the Vallejo Kaiser-Permanente Chronic Pain Program in California. Our professional partnership provided a place to develop and share ideas about how to help people-in-pain and gave me ten fruitful years to deepen my knowledge about chronic pain and its treatment.

I am grateful to have been introduced, early on, to the "client-centered" and pragmatic approach to human problems that I learned while a student at the Mental Research Institute in Palo, California. My teachers, and pioneers in the field of Brief and Family Therapy, John Weakland and Dr. Richard Fisch opened my eyes to see beyond the tinted glasses of psychiatric theory and understand the true contours of personal difficulties in their relational context. John and Dick also showed me how to relate to human problems by taking an "out-of-the-box" perspective and building strategies that lead to true problem resolution. A good deal of their approach was based on the insightful perspective of Dr. Milton M Erickson, an original thinker on human change and a masterful innovator in the field of hypnosis and psychotherapy. I am equally indebted to him and his approach to personal problems. I have also drawn from other modalities derived from Dr Erickson, including Narrative and Solution-Focused therapies.

My thinking and writing have also been influenced by the contributions of Cognitive-Behavioral and Positive Psychology researchers and practitioners as well as the work of centuries of sages and leaders from a variety of spiritual traditions. In particular, I'm indebted to the holy rabbi/master, the Baal Shem Tov ("Master of the Good Name), who wisely said "Wherever my mind is that's where I am."

The evidence base of this book was established by decades of research and clinical experience of the women and men in the chronic pain community. I especially want to thank two of these scientist-practitioners: Mark P. Jensen and David Patterson from the University of Washington. They gave me invaluable feedback and encouragement in the middle years of my writing.

There are several people whose presence on my life has been an ongoing blessing and has sustained me through this project. They include my soul brother Rabbi Avram Davis and his holy wife Laura (and let's not forget all the kids: Aliyah, Shaendl, Akiva, Zusha, and little Shirazele'). They have filled me with more family joy than one man can contain. Avram, my buddy of 40-years, has shared with me – in our "long strange trip" of life together – a quirky, solid, loving brotherhood.

Similarly, my holy soul brother and sister, Jacob and Devorah Spilman, have been amazing guiding lights for me at times when life grew dim, surprising me on so many occasions and showing me the doorway through which I entered the career of psychologist. I appreciate my friends Mark and Mona, who supported me through word and deed (and numerous overnights), your guidance and love also has sustained me in good times and bad. I also want to say Todah Rabbah ("Thanks so much") to Rabbi Eliahu Klein, Rebbetzin Cynthia and the amazing Gavi who also supported me with great gobs of family love. And thanks to the members of the Jewish Writers group in Berkeley for giving me some of my first positive critiques of this book. All I have to say to you guys is "Write on!"

I am truly grateful to the owner and staff of Morning Brew Coffeehouse and Bistro (located in Kailua, Hawai'i). My ability to write and think were significantly enhanced by the mellow and creatively stimulating environment which they manifest day after day for tourists and locals alike. I also want to thank Fred Barnett, my café colleague, a published writer, who always has a friendly "hello" and who generously shared his book preparation sources, making it possible to finally publish.

Like any good Jewish son I want to thank my mother, Lillian "Libby" Rosenbloom-Rutkay, for giving me life as well as the lively time I had living it while growing up in her house. She was a woman who suffered from a great deal of back pain yet would hardly show it, instead filling a room with laughter and good conversation. I also appreciate the copious amounts of food that she filled me and others with, and how she made sure everyone was taken care of. I miss you mom…

Last, but never least, I want to say thank-you to my beloved wife and soulmate, my Basherta ("fated one"), and girlfriend-for-life Margie Walkover who, aside from being my close friend, life partner and best love-muffin ever, edited this book in its early phases. With great intelligence, patience, and encyclopedic skill, she brought edits and structure to my creative endeavors and helped me begin the task of re-organizing content to make the book more easily useable. It goes without saying that her presence in my life is a constant, joyful and enlightening experience. Love you babe.

Little Comfort Tastes

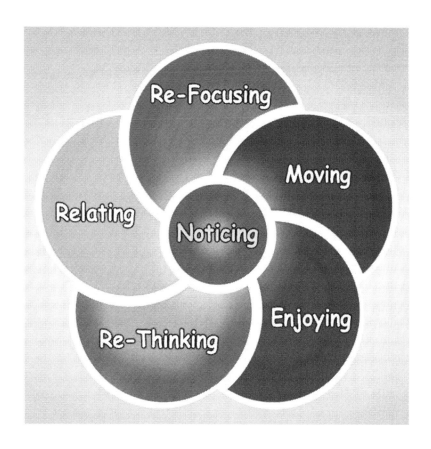

"Have You Really Tried Everything?"- A Little Story

If I ask you, "What have you done to find relief from physical discomfort?", you might respond to my question like Rob, one of my clients. He answered me by saying, "Well, I'll tell you doc – I've tried everything."

Rob suffers from severe low back pain and has found very little relief over the years. I asked him, "What have you tried?" Here is what he told me: "Well, first I went to my regular doctor and she gave me some Vicodin to kill the pain. But, after a while, I needed too much and it still didn't help enough. Then I went to see a physical therapist, but he couldn't do much. The same thing happened with a chiropractor. The next guy I saw gave me acupuncture, but that only helped a little and it didn't last long. I went back to my doctor and she sent me to a surgeon who eventually operated on me to fix my back. He promised the surgery had a very good chance of taking care of the problem. He was wrong – after three months, I started to hurt so bad that I had to take more drugs."

Unlike some people who suffer from severe pain, Rob was also willing to seek out help from psychologists who specialized in chronic pain. He said, "I went to one guy who taught me to manage the pain. It helped a little, but after a while, I just couldn't manage it - the pain was still there and that frustrated me, so I gave up. A friend of mine told me about another psychologist who was different – she told me to accept the pain and just notice it. My god! – doing that hurt like hell and I couldn't keep it up. Then I heard about this new treatment with magnets, so I..."

After listening for a while, I realized that the "everything" Rob pursued to help him feel better was actually the "same two things." First, he depended on help from a series of health professionals who offered him a variety of treatments. Second, although the techniques and treatments provided by these physicians, physical therapists, and psychologists were somewhat helpful, they all focused him on the pain – whether it was to avoid, accept, endure, or manage it.

What Rob didn't know was that there is "something else" he could do to feel better – something that could empower him to move on from pain to comfort.

Changing What Your Doctors Can't

The Best Source of Help is You

Like many people dealing with a chronic pain condition, you experience a great deal of hurt and misery. You've sought help from a whole host of medical and other professionals (i.e., doctors, surgeons, acupuncturists, chiropractors, physical therapists), and may have been surprised to discover that all the pills, shots, surgeries, and other treatments they provided have not greatly increased your comfort or happiness.

Most people seek help from a doctor when they have a medical problem. That works best for those conditions that can be fully healed. Unfortunately, chronic pain and illness are usually not curable (i.e., arthritis, Fibromyalgia, most back and neck damage). That means that repeated visits to doctors may not make much of a difference to your condition. As a "person-in-pain," when you only depend on healthcare professionals and their treatments, you're using a limited approach I call "Doctor Care Only." [1] It is disheartening that most people who struggle with chronic pain feel like they have few choices for treatment.

This brings up an important question: "What other options do you have when doctors and their treatments are not working well enough to reduce your discomfort?" The answer offered by this book is simple – *"You Have You."* If you are dealing with the problem of chronic pain, you don't have to limit yourself by only looking "out there" for a solution. The title of this book says it all – *"You are Bigger than the Pain."* This means that there is more to you than just chronic pain and misery – you have many experiences, strengths, and abilities that you can use to limit the influence of discomfort on your life. The best source of help is you and what you can do. When I tell my clients this, they usually ask me a very practical question: ***"How is it possible for me to change what my doctors can't?"*** The next section answers that question.

Pain Focusing and the Comfort Solution

Although you are the one who can make the most difference in your life, it is still necessary to consult with your doctors regarding your medical condition. You may seek treatment from physicians, medical specialists, chiropractors, acupuncturists, psychologists, or other professionals. Unfortunately, many people report that their healthcare provider has not been able to help them enough. It's quite possible that the reason is this:

Although a number of standard approaches used by your healthcare providers are helpful, their effectiveness is limited because ***they focus your attention on the pain***.

---

[1] To highlight the fact that you are a "person" dealing with ongoing pain and not merely a "pain patient," I will refer to you as a "person-in-pain."

Many pain interventions used by these professionals unintentionally direct you to focus your attention towards avoiding, accepting, or managing chronic pain. This raises your pain awareness – which may overshadow the benefits offered by your doctor.

Three approaches that are most commonly used to help people with a chronic pain condition include Traditional and some Alternative Medicine, Acceptance Therapy, and Cognitive-Behavioral Pain Management. Most practitioners of **Traditional and Alternative Medicine** encourage you to use their treatments to reduce or avoid pain and, if the treatments fail to work well enough, some doctors will tell you to "live with the pain." Those who practice **Acceptance Therapy** advise you to accept the pain and avoid doing anything to reduce it. They encourage you to notice and endure it, and develop personal values to live by. Many pain psychologists teach you **Cognitive-Behavioral Pain Management** techniques you can use to cope with and manage pain.[2] Unfortunately, all of these orientations focus you on the pain.

So, *"How is it possible for you to change what your doctors can't?"* - this book advocates something quite different → the **Personal Comfort Approach,** *which encourages you to direct your attention and efforts towards Comfort so that you'll be able to focus more on "living life" rather than "living with the pain."* (You'll find my definition of "Comfort" on the next page.) The specifics of this method, described throughout the book, are based on findings from clinical and brain-based pain research, as well as 20 years of my personal experience working with and learning from people-in-pain just like you.

Over the years, my clients' stories about improvements in their lives have taught me a lot about the relationship between pain, misery, and comfort. One key understanding is that the most powerful way to free yourself from the misery brought on by a chronic condition is to <u>allow the pain to be there while you pursue comfort</u>. Although your doctors can't do that for you, you can! (As you continue reading the book you will learn how to do that.)

A Few Core Concepts. You might ask, "What does it mean to 'pursue comfort' and how will that help me?'" The following definitions begin to answer that question:

1) **"Acute Pain"** *is the physical discomfort produced by an injury or disease that eventually fades away once the underlying medical condition heals.* It is your body's response to temporary physical damage or inflammation that creates pain signals that travel through your nervous system to the brain, causing pain, which serves as useful information telling you that your body needs some medical attention (i.e., a band-aid or a trip to the ER).

---

[2] This book re-purposes pain management skills to help you increase comfort, not focus on pain

2) **"Chronic Pain"** *is a long-term, and often constant, level of pain regularly punctuated by sharp increases in discomfort called "pain flares."* It's caused by a non-lethal – and incurable – disease, malfunction, or injury that either generates pain signals or sensitizes the brain and nervous system so that even after your body has healed from an injury or illness, you still feel pain. In other words, the original medical condition trains your brain and nerves to sense pain as if you're afflicted by an acute physical problem.

3) **"Misery"** *combines a distressed emotional state with a negative mind-set that can include depression, anxiety, anger, and stress – it's the opposite of Comfort.* It is a normal – yet unhelpful – emotional response to chronic pain and other challenging and stressful situations or people. It's usually accompanied by a mind-set of negative expectations and thoughts such a "Nothing I do will help" or "My life is over." Though it is uncomfortable, Misery is <u>not</u> physical pain. Here's how it works:

   A) Misery increases when you over-focus your attention on:
- the pain
- stressful events and annoying people
- upsetting feelings like anxiety, anger, and depression
- negative thoughts and expectations

   B) As it increases, Misery raises the sensitivity in your nervous system and that elevates your pain level. For instance, when you overly focus on the ache in your back or on depressing thoughts, you will hurt more and feel more miserable.

4) **"Comfort"** *combines a positive emotional state and optimistic mind-set that can include joy, peace, calm satisfaction, and pleasure – it's the opposite of Misery.* It helps you to positively live your life and changes your experience of pain. It allows you to feel more at ease around pain, upsetting feelings, difficult people, and other stressful situations. It can also lead to more life activity. It works in two ways:

   A) Comfort increases when you focus on:
- positive feelings and thoughts
- good experiences and people
- pleasurable activities
- optimistic expectations

   B) As it increases, Comfort desensitizes your nervous system, alters your brain, and either reduces pain or enables you to feel more at ease and comfortable around it. So how can you get more Comfort in your life? By practicing the next item.

5) **"Comfort Skills"** *are a collection of activities, exercises, and techniques that empower you to reduce Misery and increase your Comfort level.*[3] As you use these Skills, Misery is replaced by Comfort, which soothes the nervous system and reduces the influence of stress and pain.

6) **"Comfort Strategies"** *are six categories of Comfort Skills that help you to increase Comfort and solve a set of pain-related problems.* Chapter Three lists these Strategies and the Comfort Skills included in each of them.

7) **"Ownership verses Relationship."** From the perspective of this book, there are two opposite viewpoints about chronic pain:

    A) *Ownership.* Healthcare professionals, and your experience, tell you that the pain is inside of you, that it is a huge part of you and you must "own it." The problem with this "Ownership" perspective is that you cannot change an internal, incurable, chronic condition that even doctors can't repair. If you own the pain in this way, you may feel helpless or frustrated and that limits your ability to get comfortable.

    B) *Relationship.* Instead of thinking that you "have pain," imagine that you "have a relationship with pain." You can picture chronic pain as a "Bad Guy" who dominates that relationship, often weakening your sense of personal control over your life. The good news is that you can use Comfort Skills to change that relationship. Sometimes, you can even work with pain to reduce his influence.

"Who You Are Not"

Despite the discussion above, some of you may not feel like you can do anything to make a difference. In part, this may be due to feeling a loss of "self" as a result of living with chronic pain. You may either feel like you are the pain or that you don't know who you are anymore. To get back in touch with yourself, it may be useful to consider "who you are not."

---

[3] See Note #4, above.

INFO BOX #1 –
Who You are Not

❖ You are <u>not</u> imagining the pain

❖ You are <u>not</u> a complicated "head case"

❖ You are <u>not</u> a hopeless, helpless, weak victim of chronic pain

❖ You are <u>not</u> playing some pity-game to get sympathy

❖ You are <u>not</u> lazy just because you may avoid work or other activities

❖ You are <u>not</u> a desperate drug addict just because you use pain medicine

❖ And you are <u>not</u> trying to bilk insurance companies or cheat the government when you receive money they owe you

---

As a person-in-pain, you're likely to encounter unfair criticism about your situation. Perhaps some doctors, family members, friends, supervisors, or co-workers openly express doubt that you hurt or they criticize you about the changes you've had to make in your daily routine. Some people may even accuse you of being "lazy, crazy, or addicted." No matter how harsh or convincing they may sound to you, it's important to remember the facts listed in Info Box #1.

"Who You Are"

In addition to knowing "who you are not," it is also vital for your own peace of mind that you remember this:

*"You are a normal person who is dealing with a
very uncomfortable, serious, and initially debilitating condition"*

Changing What Your Doctors Can't

Once again, let's remember how you can "change what your doctor can't?" The following two actions will powerfully help you change your life for the better:

1. ***Rely on Yourself.*** *Remember that "You Have You" and, instead of looking "outside" for someone to fix you, you can look "inside" by powerfully relying on yourself to do what it takes to change your relationship with chronic pain. This can include your use of doctors' visits and treatment when it's helpful.*

2. ***Pursue Comfort.*** *An effective way to bring about change is to use your own strengths and resources along with the Comfort Skills described in this book. Together they empower you to pursue Comfort, rather than avoid, live with, blindly accept, or manage chronic pain.*

By carrying out these two actions, you will eventually feel "Bigger than the Pain." In order to help you build up a new self, Chapter Two will further orient you to the Personal Comfort Approach and compare it to "Doctor Care Only." In sum, along with moderate medical care, you can transform yourself and change a painfully hopeless existence into a life that is built on a foundation of satisfying Comfort.

"What if I Want to Start Learning the Skills Right Now?"

If you want to skip the introductory chapters and begin practicing the Comfort Skills, you can turn to Chapter Six right now and begin learning how to get more comfortable in one of the two courses described in the ***"Comfort Skills Workbook"*** (see page 69).

Why I Wrote This Book

There are two reasons why I dedicated twelve years of my life to writing this book (Okay, okay – so I'm a little slow). I first and foremost did it for those of you who wrestle with chronic pain and the problems it creates for you every day. Many of you are probably not aware that there is an option you can pursue, outside of the usual traditional or alternative medicine choices, one that will move you closer to Comfort and a happier and more satisfied life. I have a lot of experience helping people pursue that option and one of my aims is to discuss with you what Pain, Misery, and Comfort are and how you can use that knowledge to get more comfortable.

The second reason I wrote this book requires a little background. You may not know it, but the most effective way to help people-in-pain acquire some relief and a better, more meaningful, life is for them to enter an interdisciplinary "Chronic Pain Program."[4] These programs usually provide a "skills and pills" approach that combines at least three services:

1) **Mind/Body skills training and support**, taught by a Pain or Health Psychologist (these skills empower you to lower your stress and misery and raise your comfort level by changing your brain and nervous system),
2) **Moderate medical treatment**, usually in the form of medication, and,
3) **Restorative physical and occupational therapy** to build your body back into shape and balance your activity level.

Although Chronic Pain Programs are very successful in getting people back on their feet, there are very few left in this country. Over the years, they have shrunk in number from about 1000 in the late 1990s to about 150 today.[5] Many of these programs are located in university medical centers, the Kaiser-Permanente and Veteran's Administration healthcare systems, and in expensive private clinics. Because of that, most of you will not have easy access to this effective source of help.

---

[4] For resources see the American Chronic Pain Association website, http://www.theacpa.org/Pain-Management-Programs, the American Pain Society website, http://www.americanpainsociety.org/resources/content/for-people-in-pain.html, Pain.com's website, http://pain.com/pain-clinic/. and, the American Academy of Pain Management website, https://members.aapainmanage.org/aapmssa/censsacustlkup.query_page

[5] See the Institute of Medicine report, "Relieving Pain in America." Find a free digital copy online.

So?! – What is my second reason for writing this book? I want to provide you with the Mind/Body training portion of a Chronic Pain Program. Along with a moderate use of your medical provider's treatments and some physical therapy training, you can learn and use the Skills included in this training in order to get some of the benefits of an Interdisciplinary Chronic Pain Program.

What's in the Book and What is Not

The Book – A Brief Menu

Chapter One: How Does Pain and Misery Work? As the title suggests, this chapter will briefly present some of the workings of pain and how stress and emotional Misery play a significant part in how physical discomfort rises and falls.

Chapter Two: You are Bigger than the Pain – A Comfort Manifesto for People-in-Pain. Manifestos are written to challenge ineffective approaches and reveal new and better ways of doing things. In this chapter, I'm going to present two directions you can take when dealing with chronic pain: "Doctor Care Only" and the "Personal Comfort Approach." Using four questions as a guide, I'll describe the downsides of the former and the beneficial principles of the latter. In other words, I'll compare and discuss how Doctor Care Only maintains or increases your Misery and how the Personal Comfort Approach can help you build a more comfortable life.

Chapter Three: Comfort Strategies and Skills – A Descriptive List. This chapter lists the six Comfort Strategies and briefly describes the Comfort Skills included in them. It also shows you where to find them in the book.

Chapter Four: Thirteen Pain Problems and the Comfort Skills that Solve Them. These are difficulties that arise when chronic pain enters your life (i.e., poor sleep). People who want to focus their energies on solving a particular "Pain Problem" will find this short chapter helpful in locating the Comfort Skills that solve each of thirteen Pain Problems.

Chapter Five: How to Use this Book – A Few Suggestions.

Chapter Six: Workbook Introduction. This very brief chapter describes two learning styles and the two trainings included in the book, "The Brief Training," and "The Eight-Week Training."

Chapter Seven: The Brief Training. Should you decide to start with this training, you'll discover that it provides an introduction to each of six Pain Problems that can be addressed by each of the six Comfort Strategies. It also offers an additional, "bonus" Problem and Skill, which brings the total to seven. This chapter also reviews background information on each of the Problems and Skills.

Chapter Eight: The Eight-Week Basic Training. This longer program provides thirty-six Skills that you can use to solve thirteen Pain Problems. The Basic Training's eight weekly sections are divided into three "Training Days," each of which provides lessons in how to practice a set of Skills. Each Training Day offers one or more "Learn/About" segments. These briefly describe some of the background information on each Problem or Skill (see list in Appendix B).

Appendices.

- **Appendix A: Comfort Menu – Where to Find the Strategies & Skills.** A guide to locate each specific Comfort Strategy and the Skills included in them.
- **Appendix B: "Learn/Abouts" – A List of Twenty-Three.** These provide some background information on pain, Comfort, and the Comfort Skills.
- **Appendix C: Story Box List.**
- **Appendix D: Info Box List.**
- **Appendix E: Comfort Killers – Twelve Harmful Habits to Avoid.**
- **Appendix F: Useful Books & Resources for People-in-Pain.**

The Boxes

I intentionally designed this book to make it easy to use and understand. I put the most important information into a set of Boxes. My hope is that you'll be able to quickly find the content you seek by looking in one of five kinds of the Boxes.

INFO BOX #2
The Boxes

1. **Story Boxes**. Like most people, it helps me to understand problems and ideas when I can see how they manifest in the world. Storytelling is one way to bring ideas to life. I've worked with many people-in-pain over the years and I include some of their stories on these pages.

2. **Skill Boxes.** Each of these instruct you in how to use a particular Comfort Skill. They are arranged in step-by-step outline form.

3. **Contents Boxes**. These are placed at the beginning of a Training Week section and they present a "Table of Contents" specific to that week.

4. **Info Boxes.** Like the Box you are now reading, these are filled with important information, examples, and suggestions relevant to the theme of a section.

What is Not Included in this Book
Two Important Treatment Options

This book presents what I've learned from other pain experts and from the people-in-pain I've worked with over the years. That includes a large number of Skills that exercise your mind and brain and encourage you to move your body. There are at least two other approaches that help people-in-pain and are outside the scope of my training (although I work with the practitioners of these treatments). I'm certain that most of you will gain a lot from working with healthcare providers who are experts in the following areas:

1. **Functional Restoration.** When you're ready to return to physical exercise and activity, you'll benefit from working with a Physical or Occupational Therapist, Body Worker, or Exercise Trainer who'll provide treatment as well as training in how to move your body so that you get the maximum, and healthiest, amount of strengthening, balance, and flexibility possible. A moderate amount of exercise that fits your body will increase your Comfort and your daily activities.

2. **Healthy Diet.** Comfort is also enhanced by what you eat. Healthy food is good for your well-being in general, and it's especially important when you experience ongoing pain. Some pain conditions are caused or exacerbated by inflammation in the body.

The good news is that as you avoid certain foods and eat others, you will reduce some inflammatory reactions and soothe your body. Nutritionists and Naturopathic Doctors can help you discover new foods, herbs, and supplements that add to your relief.

Three More Things the Book is Not

1. **The Book is Not a Pain Psychologist.** Although it's written by a pain psychologist, the book itself is not a healthcare professional (so don't try to talk with it!). Some of you may encounter a lot of psychological or social problems and, even with the help of this program, you may still feel stuck in an uncomfortable life. In that case, I recommend that you work with a clinical psychologist who specializes in chronic pain and illness. He or she can help you figure out how to adapt the skills in this book to your particular life situation (that's what I do with my clients). Therapists can also collaborate with you on identifying stressors and learning how to overcome them. This often results in more Comfort.

2. **The Book is Not a Cure.** I wish that the training offered in these pages could take all the pain away forever and resolve the underlying condition that caused it. Alas, it can't. However, as you use this approach, you can become more comfortable than you are now. As you raise your level of positive activity and mood, you may also strengthen your Comfort and quality of life.

3. **Everything in the Book is Not Original.** Although the Comfort Approach presented in the book is original, I have adapted skills and techniques that were invented by others. I have synthesized and rearranged some of these skills and described them in a user-friendly manner. The book shares with you the fruits of decades and, in some cases, centuries (i.e., meditation) of the work and the discoveries of many people.

Introductions

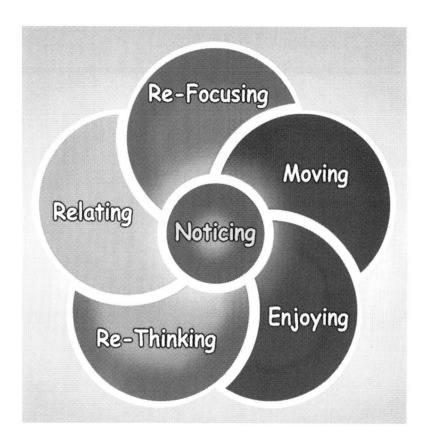

Chapter One – How Pain and Misery Work

Has anyone ever told you that the pain was "all in your head!?" Unfortunately, this insulting accusation is too often thrown in your face. Whether it's a physician, a family member, friend, or co-worker – people who say such a thing don't understand how pain works. The fact is that it's not "just mental" and you're not making it up. **"Pain"** *is experienced as an uncomfortable physical sensation, felt in one or more parts of your body, that's caused by the interaction between your mind and body and mediated by your nervous system.*[6]

So how does pain, and especially chronic pain, work? Well, it's complicated. Many years of research have revealed that the chronic pain experience is primarily due to sensory processing in your brain and nervous system, which is influenced by non-biological factors, including your personal history, mood, stress level, expectation, activites, and relationships.

This chapter will begin with a description of two types of pain. Following that, you'll learn about a very useful understanding of pain developed in the 1960s. Although it has been modified some over the years, it is still considered a major explanation of the physiology of pain. Next, you'll read about how stress alters your brain and hormonal functions and sensitizes your nervous system to experience more pain. This will include a discussion of how focusing attention on pain and negative expectations can raise your stress and discomfort levels. Finally, the section will highlight the pain-inducing effects of "Misery."

A Tale of Two Pains
Acute and Chronic

There are two types of pain: acute and chronic. Short-term or **"Acute Pain"** *is the physical discomfort produced by an injury or disease that eventually fades away once the underlying medical condition heals.* From the affected area, electrochemical pain signals arise and they move up your nervous system and register a painful feeling when they reach your brain. Although this kind of pain hurts a lot at first, the good news is that the condition that causes it will end. As it heals, the pain signals will reduce and fade away. This happened to me four years ago when I had all four of my wisdom teeth pulled. At that time, I felt a sharp ache in my jaw. Although I needed to use medication and Comfort Skills to ease some of the hurt, ten days later, the surgical wounds healed and I no longer needed to use those treatments.

"Chronic Pain" *is a long-term, and often constant, level of pain regularly punctuated by sharp increases in discomfort called "pain flares."* Unlike short-term

---

[6] See "Explain Pain" by David Butler and G. Lorimer Moseley

discomfort, chronic pain continues and is maintained by either an incurable disease, a permanent injury, unrelenting inflammation, or a repetitive nervous system cycle (i.e., CRPS/RSD). In other words, the problem with this problem is that it continues to be a problem!

Pain Hypersensitivity

"Pain Hypersensitivity" *is a state of increased sensitivity in your brain and nervous system that increases pain.*[7] This is made possible by a process called "Neuroplasticity," which is our brain and nervous system's ability to build new connections and circuits between its nerve cells. This, in turn, allows your nervous system to register ongoing pain even in the absence of bodily damage.[8] You can learn to use Comfort Skills to reverse some of that Hypersensitivity by building new Comfort connections and circuits in your brain.

Two theories developed by scientists to explain pain include the "Pain Gate Theory, and "Central Sensitization Theory." These are briefly described below.

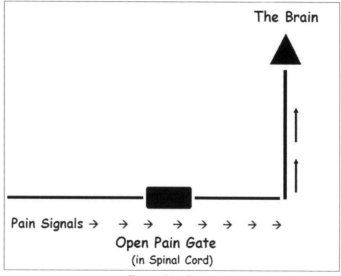

Figure #1 – Pain Gate

Theory One – The Pain Gate

Many instances of acute pain involve tissue damage and inflammation that generate pain

---

[7] See Dr Clifford Woolf's online article at
http://www.wellcome.ac.uk/en/pain/microsite/science4.html.
[8] See "Central Neuroplasticity and Pathological Pain" by Ronald Melzack & others in the Annals of the New York Academy of Sciences (2001).

signals. These pain processes are affected by stress and where you direct your attention.[9] For example, if your finger touched a red-hot stove element, the resulting damaged skin would set off an electro-chemical response that would send pain signals to your brain. Even then, these signals don't automatically shoot up into your brain. They actually have to get past a "Pain Gate" (see Figure #1, page 29).[10] In the mid-1960s, two neuroscience researchers, Melzack and Wall, discovered that a set of nerves in the spinal cord act like a gate through which pain signals must travel before they can reach the brain. Like any gate in the world, this one can temporarily open and close. When the Pain Gate closes, all or some of the pain signals are denied access to your brain. The Skills in this book help you close that Gate for periods of time.

Peripheral Sensitization

The first of two types of pain hypersensitivity comes from the parts of the body outside of the brain and spinal cord and is called "Peripheral Sensitization." Aligned with the Pain Gate Theory, it arises when your muscles and other tissues become inflamed by nearby cells that release inflammatory chemicals. These stimulate nerves that send pain signals up to the brain, causing you to feel the hurt. This includes, for example, various types of arthritis, headaches, joint problems, and muscle strains.

Theory Two – Central Sensitization

A second theory that explains chronic pain is a second type of Pain Hypersensitivity that develops in your brain and central nervous system. It is most often called "Central Sensitization." As your nerves get over-stimulated, they become abnormally excited, creating painful experiences that manifest in two different forms:

1) **Allodynia** *occurs when physical sensations that didn't hurt in the past now become irritating (i.e., a light touch on the hand).*

2) **Hyperalgesia** *happens when small pains feel like big ones (i.e., a small finger prick that feels like a stabbing knife).* The pain amplifies and lasts longer than it should.

Conditions such as Fibromyalgia, Irritable Bowel Syndrome, and certain migraine headaches may be related to Central Sensitization.

Invisible Pain

Because of hypersensitivity, many of you are treated by some family, friends, and even

---

[9] See the article, "Reconceptualising Pain According to Modern Pain Science," on Dr G. Lorimer Moseley's website, BodyInMind.org.
[10] "From the Gate to the Neuromatrix," by Ronald Melzack in the journal, "Pain" (1999).

physicians as if the pain is "in your head." This is because a number of chronic pain conditions show little physical "proof" that there is any tissue damage or other common signs of a medical impairment (i.e., Fibromyalgia). What may also cause some people to doubt you is the finding that even when there is some physical evidence, not all people feel pain. For example, in the case of Degenerative Disc Disease, only about 50% of those afflicted feel discomfort in their back. For those of you who do feel uncomfortable, the chronic pain causes more and more of your brain and nervous system to act as if your body is severely damaged, even when it is not. The result is still the same – you hurt.

Stress

Your response to emotional and physical stress also increases your sensitivity and often elevates the pain into a flare. Stressful events, such as physical overexertion, illness, depression, lack of sleep, hunger, anxiety, angry arguments, and even bad weather can further sensitize your nerves to the pain. For some time now, health researchers have known about the debilitating and destructive effects of chronic stress.[11] Two important parts of the stress process are as follows:

- **A Stressor** *is something or someone that challenges, frightens, and/or pressures you*
- **Stress** *or the* **Stress Response** *occurs when we respond to that "something or someone" with fear, anger and other negative emotions. Brings on the fight, flight or freeze reactions.*

After a person feels threatened by a Stressor, she or he will tend to jump into a "fight-flight-or-freeze" mode of action, which means that he or she will prepare to either fight off the danger, run away from it, or just stand there immobilized by fear. When this happens to you, the threat causes many things to occur in your body. Your nervous system becomes extremely aroused and it will increase your heart beat, respiration, and blood pressure, and tighten your muscles. Many researchers believe that the current epidemic of High Blood Pressure, Heart Disease, and other illnesses are due to high levels of stress. Unfortunately, the inflammatory chemical reactions and muscle tension caused by the Stress Response will also pump up your sensitivity to chronic pain.

Stress Hormone Soup

---

[11] http://www.mayoclinic.com/health/stress/SR00001 - also see the book, "Why Zebras Don't get Ulcers" by Robert Sapolsky

The Stress Response is a complicated matter in humans. Although you're not usually stressed in the same way a gazelle might be when a lion is chasing her, the challenges of modern life can stress you out and overwhelm you in other ways. One reason this happens is because your large human brain has a powerful ability to imagine and remember things. If you took thirty minutes right now and imagined that you were being chased by a lion, or that you were threatened by some other danger (i.e., losing your house), your body would respond almost like that of a frightened animal. Bad memories can also set off a stress episode. For example, if you took some time to recall your last major pain flare, you'd probably begin to feel uneasy and tense. What's worse – if you fully immersed yourself in that memory, before long, you'd sense a familiar, miserable sensation returning. If you continued to do this longer, your body might fill up with adrenaline and other stress hormones and you'd become a living bowl of "Stress Hormone Soup." Other Stressors, such as annoying supervisors, co-workers, or other difficult people, and pain itself, can set off this kind of response.

STORY BOX #1 - Stress-Free Wounds

Doctor Henry Beecher was one of the first medical professionals to recognize that physical damage did not always cause severe stress or pain. As an American surgeon, he observed an interesting phenomenon that took place in the military hospital he worked in during World War II. Many of the soldiers he worked with lost limbs or were seriously wounded in other ways. During his interviews with them, he found that only about half of them said that they were in "moderate" or "severe" pain. Even more striking was that two-thirds of that group did not request pain medicine and some even complained when the doctor tried to give them Morphine.

Dr. Beecher contrasted the soldiers' experience to that of civilian medical patients he treated some years later. These patients went through surgery while living in the United States. Even though their body damage was as severe as the soldiers' war wounds, more of the civilian medical patients were emotionally upset and complained of pain; they also asked for higher doses of pain medication. In sum, the medical patients expressed discomfort and used pain medicine more than the wounded soldiers!

Why? What was the difference between the experience of the soldiers and the surgical patients? Doctor Beecher found that the soldiers were suffering less because they focused their attention on a positive meaning for their wounds. To these soldiers, the pain meant that they would be able to outlive this war due to their injuries. They were going home! Because they concentrated on the idea that their medical condition meant "life," they did not stress out over their injuries. This idea gave them hope and increased their Comfort.

However, the peace-time surgical patients saw pain as a bad sign. To them, it was a catastrophe – they worried that they'd become disabled, lose their job, and continue to suffer. As they aimed their attention on the pain and on these negative expectations, they felt a great deal of distress, which added to their suffering and increased their use of pain medications.

Stress, Attention, and Negative Expectation

Recall that a Stressor is something that can potentially cause you to feel "stressed out." I say "potentially" because Stressors do not automatically upset you. Recall that both the soldiers and the surgical patients had serious body damage. However, many of the soldiers were not overly stressed by their wounds. The surgical patients, on the other hand, felt more stressed and uncomfortable over their injuries. Two reasons that explain the increased stress and discomfort include:

1. **Attention.** This plays a big part in stress and pain sensitivity. Here is an analogy that illustrates this: Think of an experience common to many young people During a camping trip, the kids grab a can of lighter fluid and squirt a stream of it at a campfire and watch the flames shoot up into a fireball. Similarly, when you aim your attention at a painful part of your body, usually the hurt will flare higher. When you focus your attention on pain, you build up a bigger "pain circuit" in your brain that makes you more sensitive to the hurt.

2. **Negative Expectation.** Recall that the surgical patients anticipated the worst from their medical condition and surgery. Although they directed their attention towards the pain, it wasn't just any kind of attention – it was thickly colored with *negative expectations*. Not only did these people overly focus on the pain area, but they kept

their attention fixed on a barrage of harmful ideas that interpreted the pain as an irreversible catastrophe that filled them with feelings of hopelessness, fear, despair, and frustration. It is well established that negative expectations can increase stress and pain.[12]

For example, let's say that you're moving through your day and it's been okay. Suddenly, you turn just the wrong way and your low back (or some other body part) starts to sharply ache. If you focus your attention on that part of your body you might think or say to yourself:

> "Oh damn – this is killing me! There it goes again! I can't do anything anymore; this pain is going to hurt like hell all week. What the heck am I gonna do now? I'm trapped in this misery forever…"

If this happens, you may accidentally generate in yourself a great deal of misery and that may eventually sensitize you to the pain. Like spraying a fire with lighter fluid, it will become more sharply uncomfortable. Fortunately, later in this book, you'll learn how to calm the stress, take back your attention, and let go of negative expectations. As you do that, you'll move away from physical discomfort and towards a more comfortable life.

Misery is Optional

To paraphrase a wise saying: *"Physical pain is inevitable, emotional misery is optional."* Pain is not the same as misery, although many people use the terms interchangeably. **"Misery"** *combines a distressed emotional state with a negative mind-set that can include stress, depression, guilt, rage, and anxiety.*

Here is how it works: Misery increases when you do any of the following:
- Direct your attention and thinking towards pain
- Focus on negative thoughts, expectations, perceptions, and feelings
- Overly involve yourself with people and situations that stress you out. (i.e., one woman suffered from Migraines after arguing with her husband)
- Engage in harmful or highly strenuous activities (i.e., one fellow felt more low back pain and Misery after he helped his brother move a couch)

The most important thing to remember is this: As Misery increases, the pain level goes up and that causes more Misery. This happens because negative thoughts, feelings, and actions stress your nervous system, increasing its sensitivity to chronic pain. Because Misery makes pain worse, it's important to learn how to change it. Actions that focus you on the good activities and experiences in your life reduce Misery and increase its positive opposite – "Comfort."

---

[12] See Dr G. Lorimer Moseley's article "Re-conceptualizing pain according to modern pain science."

Chapter Two – "You Are Bigger Than the Pain" – A Comfort Manifesto for People-in-Pain

Manifestos are written to challenge ineffective approaches and reveal new and better ways of doing things. This is what the American **Declaration of Independence** was all about. In this manifesto, I'm going to present two directions you can take when dealing with chronic pain: "Doctor Care Only," and the "Personal Comfort Approach." Using four questions as a guide, I'll describe the downsides of the former and the helpful principles of the latter. In other words, I'll compare and discuss how Doctor Care Only maintains or increases your Misery and how the Personal Comfort Approach can help you raise your Comfort level.

Two Approaches to Help People-in-Pain

Let's consider two sources of help you can turn to when chronic pain comes into your life. **"Doctor Care Only"** *directs you to spend much of your time passively receiving treatment from medical or other healthcare experts in a desperate effort to avoid the pain.* Most people initially choose this source because they are dealing with a medical problem. Ironically, the goal of Doctor Care Only – "avoiding the pain" – may in fact lead you to put most of your focus on pain, with little lasting relief gained from pills, spinal adjustments, or surgeries.

Even though this chapter will critique Doctor Care Only, it is important for you to remember that medical treatment is essential when you are dealing with severe acute pain, and it is somewhat helpful when you are afflicted by a chronic pain condition. You should continue to work with doctors you trust to provide useful medical treatments for your condition. However, like many of my clients, if you ONLY use these treatments, you are likely to experience very limited pain relief and lots of disappointment, two downsides of Doctor Care Only.

The **"Personal Comfort Approach"** *invites you to take charge of your life by directing your attention towards positive thoughts, feelings, actions, and experiences that will desensitize your nervous system, reduce the influence of chronic pain, and increase your Comfort.*[13] This second source of help is based on years of neuroscience and pain

---

[13] Other pain specialists also offer versions of this in the form of standard psychosocial pain management. The difference is that instead of encouraging you to manage pain, the goal of the Personal Comfort Approach is to help you increase your Comfort level around pain.

research.[14] Its name, "Personal Comfort," suggests two major differences between it and Doctor Care Only. First, it is "Personal" because you are encouraged to depend on yourself (and truly supportive others), to take charge of your body, and stand up to chronic pain. Instead of taking the passive "pain patient" role, this approach encourages you to assert your independence as a strong person-in-pain who pro-actively deals with the challenges brought on by a serious medical condition. By doing this courageous work, you will realize that you are truly *Bigger than the Pain*.

Second, the approach offered here is also about "Comfort," a soothing physical, mental, and emotional state that is the opposite of Misery and stress. When you use the skills in this book to increase your Comfort level, your nervous system will calm, and this can give you some relief. A balanced use of this approach, combined with a moderate use of medical treatments (i.e., pills), will help you regain some of your old life.

The Four Questions of Chronic Pain Care

The chart below offers four questions you can use to understand the difference between "Doctor Care Only" and the "Personal Comfort Approach." My hope is that these questions, and their answers to follow, will help you to clarify your options.

Two Approaches to Pain and Their Defining Questions		
Questions	**Doctor Care Only**	**Personal Comfort Approach**
A) What is the Goal?	❖ Avoid Pain	❖ Pursue Comfort
B) How Do You Get Help?	❖ By Depending on Doctors and Healthcare Experts (@90% of time)	❖ By Relying on Yourself and What You Can Do (@75% of time)
C) How Do You Reach Your Goal?	❖ By Only Using Medical and Other Treatments	❖ By Combining 75% Comfort Skills practice with 25% Medical Treatment
D) How Does Each Approach View Chronic Pain?	❖ Chronic Pain is Thought of as an Ownership	❖ Chronic Pain is Imagined as a Relationship

---

[14] See "The Pain Chronicles" by Thernstrom, and "A Nation in Pain" by Judy Foreman. For more on the neuroscience of brain change, see "The Brain that Changes Itself," by Norman Doidge.

Question #1 – "What is the Goal?" – Avoiding Pain versus Pursuing Comfort

"Pain Avoidance" *directs you to run away from the pain or force it out of your life using chemicals and other treatments.* This goal is central to the "Doctor Care Only" option that most of you use. It is natural, especially in the beginning stages of an acute health problem, for you to direct a lot of your attention towards the pain during medical assessments and treatments. The problem is that focusing on the problem is not very useful when it is chronic and the treatments are limited. As you'll read a little further down, there is a comfortable alternative to avoiding pain.

"Avoiding Pain" – Three Downsides
Downside #1 – Pain Avoidance Focuses You on the Pain

Pain Avoidance paradoxically focuses more of your attention and energy on the pain. One common example of this is when the doctor asks you to report your pain level on a 1-to-10 scale.[15] Another situation that makes you obsess on pain is the sole use of medication to help you avoid it. It's like you're playing a bad form of the game "Hide and Seek." When you take your medicine to "hide" from the pain, you'll "seek" it each time you check out your body to see if the pills are working. The more attention you give pain, the more you'll feel the hurt. Also, you end up concentrating on the painful part of your body as you wait the 30 to 60 minutes it takes for the pain pill to begin working. This causes many of you a great deal frustration.

Downside #2 – Pain Avoidance is Right Treatment for the Wrong Condition

Although Pain Avoidance is helpful when dealing with short-lived pain, it is minimally effective in the treatment of severe chronic pain. The vast majority of doctors are trained in the treatment of acute, short-term pain, which is brought on by a curable condition, such as appendicitis or a sprained ankle. People tolerate this kind of pain because it's caused by treatable injuries and diseases. If you have an acute condition, you're more likely to feel hope and confidence that it will heal and that you'll soon return to a normal life. Doctors freely prescribe pain medicine for such transitory problems because as you heal, you'll reduce, and eventually stop, taking pain pills. This is one reason why Pain Avoidance is a safe and effective treatment for acute pain.

The problem arises when doctors use this "right treatment" for people with the "wrong condition" – chronic pain. As chronic pain persists, many people exhaust their resources and time trying, but failing, to avoid it. Over the long run, many people-in-pain actually feel worse

---

[15] This is called the "Visual Analogue Scale" (VAS).

when doctors prescribe this acute pain treatment for their chronic condition. Pain Avoidance does not permanently reduce chronic pain or restore many of you to satisfying levels of activity. You may have to use mountains and mountains of pills for the rest of your life to escape the pain and, in the end, you won't get very far from it. Also, there is a growing national trend advising medical clinics and doctors to reduce the amount of pain medication they prescribe.[16]

Downside #3 – Pain Avoidance Increases Misery

Recall from Chapter One that **"Misery"** *combines a distressed emotional state with a negative mind-set that can include depression, anxiety, anger, and stress – it's the opposite of Comfort.* It is a normal – yet unhelpful – emotional response to personal difficulties (i.e., pain, relationship loss) that usually comes along with negative expectations and thoughts such as "Nothing I do will help" or "My life is over." When you try to out-run the pain, it often increases Misery through negative emotions, thoughts, and actions. If you make pain reduction your main goal, and the pain persists or gets worse, you're likely to feel miserable, helpless, and frustrated, which often leads to a vicious cycle of pain increasing Misery, which increases pain (see Chapter One).

"Pursuing Comfort"

Recall that **"Comfort"** *combines a positive emotional state and optimistic mind-set that can include joy, peace, calm satisfaction, and pleasure – it's the opposite of Misery.* In addition to its empowering and hopeful emotions, Comfort includes positive expectations and thoughts, such as "I can solve this" or "What a beautiful sunset."

Despite all the stereotypes, as a person-in-pain, you are not looking for more doctor appointments, pills, shots, surgeries, or diagnostic tests. Like most of the people I've worked with, what you are really seeking is ***Comfort.*** You either know, or will come to discover that, as your Comfort level rises, it will reduce the sensitivity in your nervous system to pain, helping you to move on with your life (see Chapter One).

Pursuing Comfort *invites you to simultaneously:*
1) *Allow the pain to be where it is without struggling against it or giving it a lot of attention, and instead*
2) *Direct your attention and efforts towards building up Comfort by raising your mood and cultivating a positive attitude of hope and inner strength.*

Pursuing Comfort is a powerful alternative to Avoiding Pain. The next Info Box illustrates how Misery and Comfort work.

---

[16] See American Medical Association policy on Opiate use for chronic pain.

INFO BOX #3 -
A Pillow Parable about Misery and Comfort

Imagine you are sitting in the corner of a small, locked room next to a large pile of pillows. About 15 feet away from you in the opposite corner of the room is a speaker set in the floor blasting loud, irritating music. To make things worse, it has no controls, so you can't turn it down or shut it off, and it's made out of solid steel, so you can't even break it.

At first, you get up, walk over and stand by it in order to figure out how to shut it off. Now it's really blasting in your face, and, out of frustration, you pound your fists against it, cry over it, yell at it, and give it a lot of your attention. All of these actions only increase your Misery and discomfort while the obnoxious sounds continue to blast out of that speaker.

Just before you give up all hope, you look back at the chair where you were sitting and you see the pile of pillows lying on the floor. You decide to go back there, pick up a pillow, and throw it on top of the offending speaker. To your relief, you discover that your action muffled the noise a little bit. Your ears feel a little more comfortable. Although the sound has quieted, you have not lowered the volume coming out of the speaker as it continues to scream underneath that pillow. But you don't mind because on your side of the pillow it's quieter.

You decide to pile more pillows on top of that noisy corner and, with each new pillow, you feel better and better. The annoying music sounds like it's far away even though it's going full blast below the pillows. Again, that doesn't really matter since it doesn't bother you now.

One way to think about this is that each pillow has lowered your Misery and raised up your Comfort level, regardless how loud the music plays under those pillows. In the end, you realize that the speaker can shout as much as it wants because you're feeling more comfortable <u>around</u> it.

Just as you can increase your Comfort level around an annoying speaker by covering it with pillows, you can use Comfort Skills, and your own resources, to feel more comfortable around physical pain. Even if the pain remains the same, your increased Comfort allows you to feel less irritated. These are the main goals of the Personal Comfort Approach: more Comfort and less bother.

Question #2 – "How Do You Get Help? – Over-Dependence on Doctors Versus Self-Reliance

Like you, other people-in-pain draw from one or two sources to find relief. On the one hand, Doctor Care Only leads you to seek help outside of yourself. That is, you'll be inclined to over-depend on your doctors and on other healthcare professionals to "manage" the chronic pain for you through their treatments. On the other hand, the Personal Comfort Approach and some people in the chronic pain community promote self-reliance. As I'll discuss below, when you rely mostly on yourself to bring Comfort into your life, you'll be glad that you did.

"Over-Dependence on Doctors"

Usually, when we have a medical problem, we tend to seek help "out there" from healthcare professionals. We're taught that serious sickness or pain requires consultation with medical doctors and other health experts who will determine the appropriate course of treatment. Over-dependence on doctors is appropriate when curable health problems arise, but it frequently fails to help people in chronic pain or those suffering from another chronic illness. For a while now, many of you have spent a lot of time consulting medical and alternative healthcare experts (i.e., surgeons, acupuncturists, chiropractors). For months or years, you have run after these providers and expected them to make things better. In the end, most of your doctors' efforts have provided you limited relief, and this fills you with doubt and frustration. Sadly, there is no complete solution to chronic pain "out there."

An additional problem is that *when you over-rely on doctors, you end up under-relying on yourself.* For the most part, you and the actions you take only become a very minor component of your physician's healthcare plan. Doctors work this way because they have been trained as skilled experts capable of figuring out what's wrong in order to "fix" you. Only a moderate amount of your participation in the process is needed. But when this formula fails to help, as it often does for people in chronic pain, the results can lead to more Misery and discomfort. Giving up most of the responsibility for your own care can cause you to miss out on gaining the benefit of a greater source of power and relief – YOU.

"Self-Reliance" – Four Principles

This section presents four Comfort principles that explain how relying on yourself empowers you to deal with chronic pain.

Principle One – "You've Got You"

Many of you have heard your doctors say something like: "I'm sorry, we've run out of options to treat your pain. You just have to live with it." Doctors who say this are right AND wrong. It's true that, for chronic conditions such as recurrent headaches, back and neck injuries, or Fibromyalgia, there are no medical cures. However, receiving this judgment from your doctor can feel like a dire punishment or, at the very least, a deeply frustrating piece of bad news.

Thankfully, however, being told you've run out of medical options does not mean you've reached the end of the line. That is not true. Another very effective option is still available: *You've Got You*. At first, this might sound difficult to believe. After all, what can "you" do about a medical problem like chronic pain? You're just the "helpless patient." Fortunately, at least thirty years of science has found that *You* are the best solution to the problem of chronic pain. After all, you're the one who can take back control of your mind and body by learning to practice a powerful set of skills that change your brain and increase your Comfort level.

Principle Two – "You are Responding Normally to a Real Medical Condition"

This principle encourages you to see yourself as a normal person dealing with a serious medical problem. Although this is true, your life may not feel normal. This is why, later on in the book, you'll learn how to rely more on yourself and create a "New Normal."

Principle Three – "You Are Bigger than the Pain"

Although at first it may be difficult to believe the title of this book, *"You are Bigger Than the Pain,"* it's true. That means that there is more to you than just chronic discomfort and Misery. There is a "Bigger You" who existed before pain, depression, anxiety, and other miseries came along and, as you bring that "you" out, you'll decisively decrease pain's influence on your life. One way to do this is by practicing the skills provided in the book.

Principle Four – "You Are What You Do"

When you embrace constructive action, you change who you are for the better. In fact, you can apply the idea *"You are what you do"* by taking on comfortable physical activities, new attitudes and ways of thinking, engaging in social time with good people, and re-directing your attention. These enhance your well-being and happiness. For example, you might dedicate yourself to eating healthy kinds and amounts of food, which will help you feel fit and relaxed. When it comes to chronic pain, the actions and behaviors you choose will alter your nervous system and give you the power to feel more relief and a positive mood. In other words, how you <u>act</u> directly influences how you <u>feel</u>.

Relying on Yourself – A Summary

When you rely mostly on yourself to change your relationship to pain, you bring more ease and comfort into your life without becoming over-dependent on an expert or medication. As you read on, you can receive the health information, moral support, and self-directed training that will help you to take back your life. As your skills grow, you'll rely less on doctors and other professionals, even though you may continue to need, or seek out, some of the services and remedies they offer. **The good news is that you are potentially your own best healer and best "medicine" and, with the right tools and support, you can begin to restore your health and vitality.**[17]

Question #3 – "How Do You Reach Your Goal?" – Over-Used Treatments vs. Training in Comfort Skills

The primary way that healthcare providers help you is to **do things to you**. Collectively, these things are called **"Treatment"** and they include **Medications** (chemicals that do things to you) and **Procedures** (i.e., surgery, nerve blocks). Alternative Medicine doctors, such as Chiropractors, Acupuncturists, and Naturopaths, offer their own forms of Treatment, including spinal adjustments, herbs and special diets, homeopathic remedies, magnetic procedures, etc. Often, people-in-pain end up over-relying on one or more of these Treatments. Here are four reasons why over-reliance on this option does not work in the long run.

"Over-Used Treatments" – Four Downsides
Downside #1 – "Limited Effectiveness and Availability"

In both effectiveness and availability, most Treatments for chronic pain are limited. Depending on the severity of your condition, Treatment alone will RARELY reduce the pain enough to allow you to get back to a satisfying and comfortable life.[18] On their own, high

---

[17] "Train Your Mind, Change Your Brain" by Sharon Begley; "The Brain That Changes Itself" by Norman Doidge
[18] Only two doses of pain medication will remove all the pain – 1) The first will kill you, and 2) the second turns you into a drooling zombie! Neither is very good for a happy life.

doses of pain pills, or multiple procedures such as surgery or chiropractic adjustments, will not bring most of you peace and confidence, or significantly increase your activity level. Despite all their best efforts, <u>healthcare providers and most of their Treatments are unlikely to help you any more than they already have</u>.

Although medicine may help some, when its numbing effects wear off too soon, you can't take another pill or get another shot without harming yourself. If you over-use the medication, or get too many injections in the ER, the Treatments may prove less effective over time and their availability may be limited due to a recent national trend to reduce pain medication prescriptions.

Downside #2 – "Bad Side Effects"

Another downside to Treatments is the unintended and uncomfortable effects that come along with them. The first of two of these are **"Chemical Side Effects"** brought on by medication. A sample of these include drowsiness, constipation, weight gain, poor concentration, and sexual problems. In addition, some Treatments may harm you if over-used (i.e., Opiates). Some of you may have taken quantities of medicine to the point where your life was in danger and you were rushed to the ER to get your stomach pumped. Death from over-use is the worst side effect and it happens too often.

"Failed Procedures" are a second type of bad side effect. These include malfunctioning Spinal Stimulators and Opiate Implants, which can cause infection. Although they do offer some pain relief, research shows that they have little effect on raising your activity level.[19] Another Failed Procedure includes some back surgeries (i.e., fusions), which have an even worse track record, and may create more pain. Many of you understandably had high expectations that surgery would solve the medical problem and, when it didn't, you lost hope and felt terrible. All of the broken promises made by some well-intentioned surgeons made things worse.

Downside #3 – "Negative Psychological Effects"

Two additional non-physical problems arise when you over-rely on pain Treatments. These negative psychological consequences affect how you "view and do" things in relation to chronic pain (see next Info Box).

---

[19] See the book, "Chronic Pain: An Integrated Biobehavioral Approach" by Herta Flor and Dennis Turk.

INFO BOX #4 –
Two Negative Psychological Effects

1. **Passivity and Frustration.** Over-use of Treatments makes you a passive recipient of medical advice and therapies, which often leads to feelings of helplessness and loss of control. Over-use of medicine, like doctor over-dependence, also lessens your sense of responsibility and capacity to care for yourself in other ways. You also become frustrated when the medicine does not work well enough. Some of you may believe the hopeless idea that no other source of help exists. (This book was written to butt-kick that belief!!)

2. **Fruitless Searching for the Perfect Treatment.** You might have the habit of running around looking for the cure. If you keep searching for the "Right Treatment," after it's clear that there are none, you'll feel more miserable and frustrated, and you won't move on in your life.

Downside #4 – "High Cost of Health Care"

Need I say more – when the only source of help you seek is from the Medical and Alternative Healthcare System, you will most likely spend a great deal of money on finding relief. This may include high health insurance deductibles and co-pays, the high cost of medications and procedures, or out-of-pocket spending on outside practitioners that your insurance will not cover.

"Training in Comfort Skills" – Four Principles

As suggested in the "Pillow Parable" (see Info Box #3, page 39), you can reduce Misery and even physical discomfort by learning how to get more comfortable around the pain. Remember, Comfort is a "pleasant state of body and mind that puts you at ease, fills you with a sense of calm and confidence, and may produce feelings of pleasure." It is the opposite of Misery and increases when you a) focus on positive feelings and thoughts, b) focus on the good people around you, and (c) focus on pleasurable activities. By learning how to raise your Comfort, you can attain a satisfactory level of calm and relief. The following four principles describe how this Training does this.

Principle #1 – Comfort Skills and Strategies

"Comfort Skills" *are a collection of activities, exercises, and techniques that empower you to reduce Misery and increase your Comfort level.* Practicing them is an alternative to passively over-depending on doctors and treatments. Pain specialists and researchers developed these Skills over many years.[20] Some practices come from traditional cultures (i.e., meditation) and others were discovered and developed by clinical and academic researchers (i.e., mood and thought changing techniques).[21] Other Comfort Skills come from common sense, such as pacing your activities in order to avoid the overdoing that leads to pain flares (i.e., lifting heavy objects).

Most professionals call these Skills "pain management" or "pain coping techniques." As described earlier, I am re-purposing these Skills to help you increase your Comfort, not manage-avoid-accept-control pain (see Question One, above). When you practice Comfort Skills, you actually restructure the brain and desensitize your nervous system, which either reduces pain or makes it easier to deal with. The Skills also help you to dissolve Misery and increase your activities. They empower you to rely more on yourself than on professionals.

"Comfort Strategies" *are six categories of Comfort Skills that help you to increase Comfort and solve a set of pain-related problems.* The workbook sections in this book (Chapters Six, Seven and Eight) will introduce you to these Strategies, which include **Noticing, Re-Focusing, Moving, Enjoying, Re-Thinking, and Relating**. They are graphically represented on a "Comfort Wheel" (see Figure #2, below). Also, Chapter Three provides you a brief introduction to all the Comfort Strategies and the Skills they contain.

Principle #2 – "It Only Works When You Work It"

There is one "catch" to the effectiveness of the Comfort Skills – you need to practice them in order to experience benefits. *It only works when you work it.* This is a no-brainer – when you use a tool, it helps you fix what needs fixing. If you don't use it, nothing gets fixed. The Skills offered in this book could repair some of what is broken in your daily life. However, in order for that to happen, you need to take the time and make the effort to practice. Many of the people who made and kept their commitment to learn and use these Skills discovered they had more control over distress and discomfort than they had first thought.

---

[20] "A Nation in Pain," by Judy Foreman
[21] "Psychological Approaches to Pain Management: A Practitioner's Handbook," - Dennis Turk & Robert Gatchel

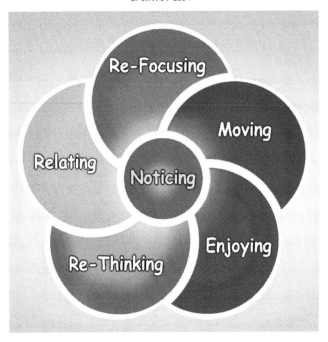

Principle #3 – Balancing "Skills and Pills"

Instead of limiting your choices by recommending that you <u>only</u> use medicine or <u>only</u> practice Comfort Skills, this approach encourages you to use a healthy balance of both. Eventually, a number of you may feel so good that you will choose to use fewer pills than Skills. (If you decide to do that, be sure to work with your doctor to carefully reduce your medications.)

Principle #4 – "Good Side Effects"

Most people who use the Skills to pursue Comfort experience no bad side effects. On the contrary, the results are very good and include increased positive mood, better sleep or rest, higher confidence, more activity, and reduced pain flares and/or better toleration of discomfort. This principle encourages you to notice and remember these positive effects.

Question #4 – "How Does Each Approach View Chronic Pain?" - Ownership vs. Relationship

There are two well-established medical viewpoints that are applied to chronic pain. The **Biomedical Approach**, which is followed by most physicians, surgeons, and other traditional healthcare providers, understands pain as a biological problem that can only be effectively controlled through chemical, surgical, or other Treatments. Another perspective, promoted in this book, rests on a relatively new evidence-based healthcare orientation called the **Biopsychosocial Approach**.[22] The doctors, psychologists, medical social workers, and other practitioners who work within this modality take into account the physical, psychological, and social influences that affect illness and healing.

You can think about these two viewpoints as representing an **"Ownership"** of, or a **"Relationship"** with, the pain condition. Although both offer solutions to the problem of chronic pain, this book considers the Relationship Approach as more empowering and effective.

"Pain as an Ownership"

"Ownership" *is a perspective that defines chronic pain as a condition that you have.* Most of you have been taught to believe that the pain condition is inside of you and that you have to "own" it and tell others that "it's my pain." Consequently, like any other physical problem, you'll believe that it's part of you and belongs to you. This logically follows from the assumptions of the Biomedical approach practiced by most medical professionals, and from your own common sense and experience of the pain feeling inside of you.

When Ownership is Helpful – Acute Pain

The Ownership approach is absolutely necessary when it comes to treatable conditions that cause acute pain. For example, if you broke your leg, it makes sense for you to think of it as "my broken leg" and to experience the acute pain that comes from that injury as "my pain." In order to feel better, you'll seek medical help to help you return to heath. You'll also focus your attention on the leg's short-term pain during the healing process to identify the signs that tell you the leg is healing. When the acute pain eases, you'll know the leg is getting better, and, when it heals, you'll no longer "have" pain.

When Ownership is Not Helpful – Chronic Pain

The difference between acute and chronic pain illustrates how owning the latter is not helpful. As stated above, the signals given out by acute pain let you know that something is broken and needs fixing. However, the signals sent out by chronic pain, at best, usually communicate that the pain area has been irritated, **not** that more damage is occurring.[23] In other words, *"It's not an emergency, it just hurts!"* Many of you may read chronic pain signals as acute pain signals, because they can feel the same. You may think you're

---

[22] See the journal article by George I Engel, "The need for a new medical model: The challenge of biomedicine," in Science, April 8, 1977, Volume 196, Number 4286, pages 129-136.
[23] Of course, if something like a car accident comes along to further damage the area, you will feel both Acute and Chronic Pain

experiencing a physical problem that needs immediate medical attention, causing you to run to a physician or Emergency Room. Once there, the doctor may say "there is nothing much that can be done to repair this problem." This kind of assessment can upset you and increase your Misery.

Others of you who believe that a pain flare is warning you about new damage might become vulnerable to false hopes provided by some well-meaning (or some unscrupulous) healthcare providers who claim that their procedure or remedy will "cure the problem inside of you" or "make it a lot better." You might believe this even after numerous, competent doctors have already told you that there is no cure. When "new" Biomedical or Alternative Medicine procedures fail to heal you, you're likely to fall deeper into despair or depression. This further reinforces the thought that you are stuck with owning this pain that is stuck inside of you.

"Pain as Relationship"

Instead of "having pain," it is possible to think about it in a different and more empowering way. **"Relationship"** *is a perspective that invites you to imagine that you have a relationship with pain.* This viewpoint is based on the Biopsychosocial approach and recognizes the influence of physical, social, and psychological factors on illness. However, I will take this idea a step further by inviting you to think about your chronic pain experience quite differently. First, remove from your shoulders the burden of Pain Ownership and consider the idea that the source of pain is outside of you. One way to do this is to imagine is a "Bad Guy" outside of you who sends uncomfortable feelings into your body, and fills your mind with negative thoughts that focus you on painful sensations and upsetting ideas (i.e., "This will never stop!"). Therefore, instead of thinking about pain as an Ownership, imagine that it's a Relationship (and pain often dominates that relationship). This new perspective also encourages you to stand up as well to chronic pain's destructive "buddies" → Depression, Stress, Anxiety, Guilt, and Rage.

"Two Empowering Action Ideas"

The viewpoint described above is succinctly summarized in a set of two "Empowering Action Ideas." An **"Action Idea"** *is a concept that you can act on.* In the next Info Box, you'll find a brief description of these Action Ideas.

INFO BOX #5 –
Two Empowering Action Ideas

1. **You are not the pain, pain is the pain.** To paraphrase J.C. Duggart (a young woman who survived kidnapping and captivity), "the pain isn't who you are, it's only what happens to you." Too often, you or others may get the impression that your life is all about pain. You may take on the myth that "you are the pain problem" or that the pain is something deeply connected to you on the inside. As you focus on the truth that you're not the pain, you will begin to separate yourself from it.

2. **You can use Comfort Skills to change your relationship with pain.** When you see pain as a Bad Guy, it's easy to act as if you have a "Relationship" with "him." It's not the relationship you want and it often feels like pain dominates it. However, like many individuals, you have learned how to improve your relationships with people, yourself, and challenging situations. Because of this, you can use your own abilities, along with Comfort Skills, to take more control of your Relationship with chronic pain. This places you more in charge of your brain, your body, and your life. You can also act as if you have a Relationship with pain's "buddies" (Depression, Anxiety, Rage, and Stress) and change them as well.

When you think about pain as a Relationship, you're better able to stand back and observe all of the physical, psychological, and social influences within and around you that alter the discomfort. For example, let's say that you get flared and your spouse, or another family member, nags you about "not being more active." If this upsets you, you're likely to feel more Misery and pain. When they nag you, it may seem as if they are "working with pain and Misery against you." Sadly, they may not know it, but their behavior makes you more vulnerable to pain. You can stop this unhelpful pattern by using some of the Relating Skills to set limits on their verbal intrusion (see page 59). By imagining that pain is a Relationship, you can empower yourself to change it.

Ownership vs. Relationship – A Final Note

Obviously, you are free to think about pain any way you wish. In fact, you can practice the Comfort Skills in this book and feel better whether or not you believe you Own or Relate with Pain. For example, some people believe that food is a luscious experience that they must have and they tend to put a lot of effort into cooking or choosing good restaurants. Other people, however, think of food as a necessary inconvenience and will cook easy things or grab a quick bite somewhere. Regardless of which way food is conceived, both groups of people are eating and getting nourished. Similarly, whether you choose to imagine that pain is something that you have or relate with, the most important idea to remember is that when you regularly use Comfort Skills, and your own resources, you can make a positive difference in your life.

Chapter Three – Comfort Strategies & Skills – A Descriptive List

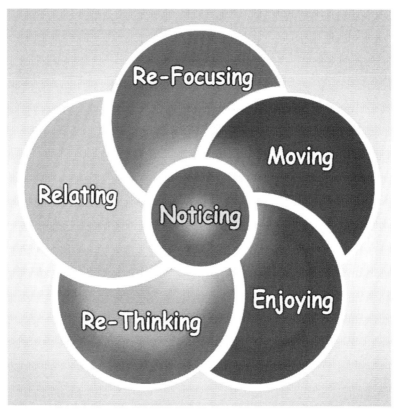

The Comfort Wheel

Six Comfort Strategies Changing Your Relationship to Pain

The Comfort Skills are organized into Six "Comfort Strategies" (see Comfort Wheel above). Remember, **"Comfort Strategies"** *are six categories of Comfort Skills that help you to increase Comfort and solve a set of pain-related problems.* This chapter will show you the Comfort Skills included in each Comfort Strategy.[24]

---

[24] You can also find page numbers for each Comfort Skill training box in Appendix A, on page 338.

INFO BOX #6 –
"The Six Comfort Strategies"

First Strategy – NOTICING. Before you can solve a problem, it's helpful to see it first - that's why Noticing is in the center of the Wheel. The first of two Skills shows you how to identify "Negatives" that either set off or warn you about a coming pain flare or emotional upset. Two other Noticing Skills shine your awareness on the "Positives" that improve your day (i.e., more sleep) or on new changes in your situation now compared to the past.

Second Strategy – RE-FOCUSING. This set of Skills help you redirect your attention away from pain and towards something neutral or pleasant. Each Re-Focusing practice potentially relaxes your mind and body and reduces stress and sensitivity in your nervous system. These include Positive Distraction, Breathing Techniques, Meditation, Imagery, and Self-Hypnosis.

Third Strategy – MOVING. This strategy shows you how to comfortably and effectively move through four important events in your life: Moving the Body, Goal Setting, Sleep and Rest, and Pain Flares.

Fourth Strategy – ENJOYING. More than most people, you deserve a great deal of pleasure and joy in your life. The good news is that you can have it, even if pain comes along for the ride! What's even better is that when you use Enjoying Skills to generate pleasure your mood will improve and pain will take a back seat. This Strategy includes Laughter, Fun, Positive U-Turns (away from bad situations), and Positive Qualities (i.e., Gratitude, Generosity).

Fifth Strategy – RE-THINKING. You may have noticed that low moods, anxiety, stress, and pain-focusing are often brought on by Negative Thoughts. For example, if you follow the thought, "My life is over," it may take you down to despair. This Strategy includes three Re-Thinking Skills that enable you to prevent bad thoughts from turning into depression, panic, anger or pain. This Strategy also includes a Skill to improve your memory.

Sixth Strategy – RELATING. Your physical and emotional Comfort is profoundly impacted by your interactions with people. Pain and Misery levels rise when you isolate yourself from good people, argue a lot, or give in to the criticisms or manipulations of annoying people. Conversely, when you spend time with friendly people, avoid arguments, and use Relating Skills to set firm limits on annoying people, you'll feel stronger, calmer, and more at ease.

First Comfort Strategy – Noticing

Noticing Skill Solutions – Negatives
Noticing Skill # 1 – "Revealing Triggers"

This Noticing Skill shows you how to identify "negatives" in your life. These **"Triggers"** *are people or situations that set off a bad mood or a pain flare* (i.e., bright lights, a yelling spouse). They usually originate outside of you, in the physical or social world, or from an activity (see Chapter 8, Week Two, First Training Day, page148).

Noticing Skill # 2 – "Revealing First Signs"

A second set of Negatives are **"First Signs,"** *which take place inside your body and mind and warn you that a pain flare or emotional upset is coming.* For example, muscle tension, negative thoughts and images, upset emotions, or harmful habits (i.e., over-eating). First Signs are often a response to a Trigger. Both Triggers and First Signs alert you to do something to prevent a painful episode (see Chapter 8, Week Two, First Training Day, page 149).

Noticing Skill Solutions – Positives
Noticing Skill #3 – "I Want to See More of…"

"Positives" *are satisfying changes and events that increase your comfort and well-being.* This is the first of two Noticing Skills that shows you how to observe what's going well. It trains you to track the good things that arise in your life (even small ones). (See Chapter 8, Week Two, Second Training Day, page 165.)

Noticing Skill #4 – "Comparison Questions"

After completing part or all of the Trainings in this book, and practicing the Skills you've learned, many of you will notice some improvements happening in your daily life. The questions provided in this last Positive Noticing Skill help you see what is positively different now compared to where you were in the past. (See Chapter 8, Week Two, Second Training Day, page 322.)

Second Comfort Strategy – Re-Focusing Skills

Re-Focusing Skill #1 – "Breath Count"

The title says it all – this Skill instructs you to count each exhale quietly in your mind. After you reach ten breaths, start over again with "one." Like the other Re-Focusing Skills, when you notice that you've gotten distracted by thoughts, sounds or feelings, gently return your attention back to the breath and the count. (See Chapter 8, Week One, First Training Day, page 130.)

Re-Focusing Skill #2 – "Breath Massage"

This practice enables you to "massage" your body by imagining that your breath is flowing through each body part. As you focus intently on it, you may begin to feel like you're receiving a massage. (See Chapter 8, Week Two, Second Training Day, page 151.)

Re-Focusing Skill #3 – "Mantra/Breath Meditation"

The first of two Meditation techniques described in this book, "Mantra/Breath Meditation," allows you to alter how your brain processes pain signals and it strengthens your ability to focus your attention. (See Chapter 8, Week Three, Second Training Day, page 198.)

Re-Focusing Skill #4 – "Mindfulness Meditation/Thought Labeling"

This is one form of a powerful method to reduce suffering and raise your Comfort. It was introduced to the medical world by Dr. Jon Kabat-Zinn, a research scientist in the early 1980s. As you practice this style of Meditation distractions will bother you less, your mind and nervous system will become calmer, and your body will feel more at ease. (See Chapter 8, Week Four, Second Training Day, page 226.)

Re-Focusing Skill #5 – "The Head Trip"

Daydreaming is a kind of "skill" that we all use when we're bored or just want to fantasize about something. In a way, when you use your imagination to go on a "Head Trip," your body may pleasantly surprise you. (See Chapter 8, Week Five, Second Training Day, page 245.)

Re-Focusing Skill #6 – "Self-Hypnosis – Three Inductions"

These hypnotic techniques invite you to choose from three options that enable you to move into a trance-like state of relaxation. (See Chapter 8, Week Seven, Third Training Day, page 311).

Re-Focusing Skill #7 – "Positive Distraction – The Fast and Slow Menus"

Research and common sense have shown that when you distract yourself, you temporarily forget what you were experiencing in the moment. Positive Distractions may interrupt the pain, even for a little while. There are two forms of this Skill suggested in Chapter 8, Week Six, Second Training Day, page 265.

Re-Focusing Skill #8 – "Immerse in a Good Memory"

This Skill combines the internal concentration that characterizes Re-Focusing Skills with the pleasant feeling brought about by Enjoying Skills. It is the practice of replaying wonderful memories in your mind and fully re-experiencing and enjoying them. (See Chapter 8, Week Four, Third Training Day, page 230.)

Third Comfort Strategy – Moving Skills

Goal Setting
Moving Skill #1 – "Set a Goal, Create a Future"
Often, when chronic pain or Depression comes along, you may feel like you have no future. You might Under-Do your activity by lying around too much (this usually makes things worse over time). When you set a goal, (i.e., social, exercise, work), you're telling Depression and Pain that you <u>do</u> have a future. You'll also return to a balanced level of activity and build a new life, goal by goal. There is no rush – the practice works best when you go at a slow, steady pace by taking "Baby Steps" – that is, move one small step at a time. (See Chapter 8, Week One, Second and Third Training Days, page 133 & 138.)

Moving the Body
Moving Skill #2 – "Pay as You Go"
Many people in pain tend to Over-Do their activities beyond what their body can comfortably handle. If you want to avoid pain flares brought on by over-exertion and high stress, use this Skill to adjust a task so that it fits your body and increases Comfort. (See Chapter 8, Week Two, Third Training Day, page 169.)

Moving Skill #3 – "The Payment Plan."
For those of you who believe that Over-Doing a certain activity is worth the pain flare you'll get, there is still an option you can use to effectively cope with the increased discomfort. The three components of this Skill will enable you to more easily handle a pain flare and, in the end, you may ride it out more comfortably than in the past. (See Chapter 8, Week Two, Third Training Day, page 176.)

Sleep and Rest
Moving Skill #4 – "Day Skills for Night Sleep"
When you use some or all of this collection of techniques during the day, you can improve your ability to sleep at night. (See Chapter 8, Week Three, First Training Day, page 184.)
Moving Skill #5 – "Rest in the Bed"

This is one of two powerful Skills you can use if you have a difficult time falling and/or staying asleep. When you follow its three steps, you can feel more rested in the morning, even if you did not sleep that night. (See Chapter 8, Week Three, First Training Day, page 186.)

Moving Skill #6 – "Working Back to Bed"

If you find it difficult to stay in bed at night when you can't sleep, this second night-time Skill gives you a work assignment that can lead you back to a bed of sleep or rest. (See Chapter 8, Week Three, First Training Day, 188.)

Moving Through a Pain Flare

Moving Skill #7 – "Flare Planning in Sets of Three"

When pain flares come along, this Moving Skill helps you to more effectively ride them out. It will instruct you on how to set up a plan to deal with future increases in pain. (See Chapter 8, Week Six, Third Training Day, page 270.)

Moving Skill #8 – "Two Bottles of Comfort"

There are two bottles you can use to help you handle a pain flare. The "Skill Bottle" is a device that increases your recall of those Skills that help you deal with chronic pain. The second, The "Flare Bottle" offers you a safe way to use short-acting opiates and other pain medications to help you increase your Comfort during a pain flare. In consultation with your doctor, you may find that using this Skill will enable you to use your medication more effectively. (See Chapter 8, Week Sid, Third Training Day, page 273.)

Fourth Comfort Strategy – Enjoying Skills

Enjoying Right Now

Enjoying Skill # 1 – "Laughing"

This Skill invites you to bring more Laughter into your daily life. There is ample medical and psychological evidence that laughter raises your Comfort level and contributes to your general health (laugh right now and see what happens). As long as laughter does not irritate the part of your body that hurts, you'll notice that when you use this Skill, you'll feel lighter, happier, and more at ease. (See Chapter 8, Week Two, Second Training Day, page 158.)

Enjoying Skill # 2 – "Doing Fun"

Similar to Laughing, this lifestyle practice raises your mood and makes it easier to tolerate physical pain. Pleasurable activity does not have to be expensive or even strenuous. The important point of this Skill is to increase the times in your life when you are enjoying yourself, even a little. (See Chapter 8, Week Two, Second Training Day, page 162.)

Positive U-Turn
Enjoying Skill #3 – "Counter a Negative with a Positive"

This Enjoying Skill helps you to "snatch joy from the mouth of Misery." When you're in a painful situation, you may often feel like you are trapped and that there's no escape. Use this Skill to counter a Negative that's in your face and you may be surprised at the joy that pops out! (See Chapter 8, Week Five, First Training Day, page 239.)

Cultivating Positive Qualities
Enjoying Skill #4 – "Write a Gratitude Letter"

A **"Positive Quality"** *is a strongly held, life affirming purpose, value, and ability that defines your character.* Recently, scientists have identified twenty-four of these.[25] One of the most powerful Positive Qualities is "Gratitude." When you engage in it, you have the potential to develop a sense of appreciation for life - something very difficult to do when dealing with chronic pain. (See Chapter 8, Week Five, Third Training Day, page 253.)

Enjoying Skill #5 – "Filling a 'Good Stuff' Journal"

Another way to cultivate your Quality of Gratitude is to keep a Journal dedicated to the "Good Stuff" in your life. (See Chapter 8, Week Five, Third Training Day, page 254.)

Fifth Comfort Strategy – Re-Thinking Skills

Re-Thinking Memory
Re-Thinking Skill #1 – "Look in the Book"

Since memory loss and poor concentration are common in people who are in chronic pain, you will find it most useful to take on this Re-Thinking Skill. (See Chapter 8, Week Three, Third Training Day, page 205)

Re-Thinking Negative Thoughts

---

[25] See Christopher Peterson and Martin Seligman's boo, "Character Strengths and Virtues: A Handbook and Classification" 2004.

Re-Thinking Skill #2 – "See it Coming"

Pain, Depression, and other "Bad Characters" often send Negative Thoughts into your mind when you feel emotionally vulnerable and physically uncomfortable. Thoughts like "My life is over" or "I'm just a cripple" will usually bring your mood down or worry you and this causes the pain and Misery to rise. This Re-Thinking Skill shows you how to *catch these thoughts before they catch you*, enabling you to stand up to them, build your self-control, and raise up your mood. (See Chapter 8, Week Four, First Training Day, page 215.)

Re-Thinking Skill #3 – "Re-Mind Yourself About the Truth"

Just like a number of lawyers and politicians, Negative Thoughts lie to you. Untruths such as "you're a loser," or "you are a lazy burden on everyone" can really hurt you if you believe them. This Skill reminds you to consider what is true when such harmful thoughts come along. (See Chapter 8, Week Four, First Training Day, page 218.)

Re-Thinking Skill #4 – "Talk Back and Step Aside"

When Negative Thoughts bug you, you'll find it very helpful to "talk back" to them in your mind. When you do this, and combine it with "stepping aside" (distracting yourself), you'll weaken that thought and improve your mood. This prevents additional pain and suffering that often accompanies people in pain who fall into depression or anxiety. (See Chapter 8, Week Four, First Training Day, page 220.)

Sixth Comfort Strategy – Relating Skills

Relating with Good People

Relating Skill #1 – Build New Relationships with Old Friends and Family

Many people in pain are socially isolated and feel very, very lonely. This Relating Skill shows you how to renew old relationships with the good people in your life. Most social and health scientists agree that positive relationships lead to positive feelings and physical health. (See Chapter 8, Week Six, First Training Day, page 260.)

Relating Skill #2 – How to Meet New Friends

New relationships also increase your joy. Some of you may have noticed that when you've been abandoned by some of the people in your life you discover who your real friends are. The goal of this second Relating Skill is to help you explore new people who might turn into true friends. (See Chapter 8, Week Six, First Training Day, page 262.)

Dealing with Annoying People Directly

Relating Skill #3 – "The C.A.L.M. Nice Guy Approach"

Many of us have "Annoying People" in our lives. These are usually loved ones or co-workers who annoy you from time to time or bother you about a particular issue (i.e., spending money, use of pain medication). There are also "Seriously Annoying People" – those who irritate you most every day (i.e., a sarcastic, controlling spouse). Whether they bother you a little or a lot, the result is the same – you feel stressed out, miserable, and pained. When you set an effective limit on their behavior, especially on their hurtful words, your life will feel much better. The "C.A.L.M. Nice Guy Approach is one direct method to say "No!" to an Annoying Person. (See Chapter 8, Week Seven, First Training Day, page 290.)

Relating Skill #4 – "The C.U.T. Tough Guy Approach"

This is another direct way to say "No!" to an Annoying Person. The "C.U.T. Tough Guy Approach" shows you how to immediately get firm with those who don't respect your reasonable requests. (See Chapter 8, Week Seven, First Training Day, page 294.)

Dealing with Annoying People Indirectly

Relating Skill #5 – "One Down Duck Down"

Some situations call for a more indirect approach to say "No!" to the abuses of Annoying People. The "One Down Duck Down" is quite effective in stopping the verbal abuse and preventing yourself from getting defensive. (See Chapter 8, Week Seven, Second Training Day, page 297)

Relating Skills #6 – "Disarm Them in the F.O.G."

This technique gives your tormentors an indirect consequence for the irritation they cause you. Often, that will dissuade them from bothering you in the future. (See Chapter 8, Week Seven, Second Training Day, page 298.)

Relating Skills #7 – "Distracted Listening"

Don't you wish you could find a way to avoid listening to an Annoying Person spouting his or her hurtful, irritating words? This Skill shows you how to indirectly set a limit on their Toxic Talk by getting distracted on purpose (See Chapter 8, Week Seven, Second Training Day, page 301.)

Chapter Four – Thirteen Pain Problems and the Comfort Skills that Solve Them

Introduction

As you know quite well, chronic pain, all by itself, is a serious problem. Unfortunately, it also causes "**Pain Problems**," *which are pain-related difficulties that increase your Misery* (and eventually increases your hurt). They include common troubles such as poor sleep and low moods. Researchers and clinical professionals know that if these problems are left unsolved, they can exacerbate or maintain Misery and pain levels (i.e., a poor night's sleep results in an uncomfortable day).

The next Box contains thirteen common Pain Problems. The balance of this chapter presents a brief description of each Pain Problem and the Comfort Skills that can solve it (see "Appendix A" to locate the page for each Comfort Skill).

INFO BOX #8 –
"Thirteen Pain Problems that Accompany Chronic Pain"

1. Unpredictable Pain Flares and Emotional Distress

2. Attention Hijacked by Pain and Stress

3. Poor Sleep and Rest at Night

4. Sadness, Worry, and Other Miserable Feelings

5. Negative Thoughts

6. Distress Caused by Annoying People

7. Underprepared for Pain Flares

8. Missing the Good Things in Your Life

9. Hypersensitive Nervous System

10. No Positive Future in Sight

11. Unbalanced Activity

12. Poor Memory

13. Isolation and Loneliness

Pain Problem #1 -
"Unpredictable Pain Flares and Emotional Distress"

Difficulties like pain flares and emotional upsets seem to come out of nowhere, leaving you feeling helpless and frustrated.

- Noticing Skill #1 – "Revealing Triggers"
- Noticing Skill #2 – "Revealing First Signs"

Pain Problem #2
"Attention Hijacked by Pain and Stress"

Your attention becomes overly absorbed by pain as well as stress, anxiety, and/or other emotional upsets. This is because you have unknowingly allowed yourself to focus on these difficulties and your brain has grown used to directing its attention towards them.

- Enjoying Skill #1 – "Laughing"
- Enjoying Skill #2 – "Doing Fun"
- Enjoying Skill #3 – "Counter a Negative with a Positive"

- Re-Focusing Skill #1 – "Breath Count"
- Re-Focusing Skill #2 – "Breath Massage"
- Re-Focusing Skill #3 – "Mantra/Breath Meditation"
- Re-Focusing Skill #4 – "Mindfulness/Thought Labeling Meditation"
- Re-Focusing Skill #5 – "The Head Trip"
- Re-Focusing Skill #6 – "Self Hypnosis – Three Inductions"
- Re-Focusing Skill #7 – "Positive Distraction: The Fast and Slow Menus"
- Re-Focusing Skill #8 – "Immerse in a Good Memory"

Pain Problem #3
"Poor Sleep and Rest at Night"

You feel exhausted and achy in the morning because you had a difficult time falling and/or staying asleep. In part, this is because you're dealing with many distractions, physical and psychological, that keep you awake.

- Moving Skill #4 – "Day Skills for Night Sleep"
- Moving Skill #5 – "Rest in the Bed"
- Moving Skill #6 – "Working Back to Bed"

Pain Problem #4 –
"Sadness, Worry, and Other Miserable Feelings"

You find little pleasure in life and often feel depressed, angry, worried, anxious, and/or bored. These feelings are often brought on by the uncomfortable sensations you feel in your body. These miseries make it difficult for you to feel pleasure or anything good.

- Re-Focusing Skill #1 – "Breath Count"
- Re-Focusing Skill #2 – "Breath Massage"
- Re-Focusing Skill #3 – "Mantra/Breath Meditation"
- Re-Focusing Skill #4 – "Mindfulness/Thought Labeling Meditation"
- Re-Focusing Skill #5 – "The Head Trip"
- Re-Focusing Skill #6 – "Self Hypnosis – Three Inductions"
- Re-Focusing Skills #7 – "Positive Distraction: The Fast and Slow Menus"
- Re-Focusing Skill #8 – "Immerse in a Good Memory"
- Enjoying Skill #1 – "Laughing"
- Enjoying Skill #2 – "Doing Fun"

- Enjoying Skill #3 – "Counter a Negative with a Positive"
- Enjoying Skill #4 – "Write a Gratitude Letter"
- Enjoying Skill #5 – "Filling a 'Good Stuff' Journal"

Pain Problem #5
"Negative Thoughts"

You're plagued by negative thoughts that relentlessly drive you into emotional distress and harmful habits – both of which tend to increase pain. This is because your situation often brings on these thoughts and you unknowingly follow them down the road to miserable places.

- Re-Thinking Skill #2 – "See it Coming"
- Re-Thinking Skill #3 – "Re-Mind Yourself About the Truth"
- Re-Thinking Skill #4 – "Talk Back and Step Aside"

Pain Problem #6
"Distressed by Annoying People"

There are people in your life that you relate with regularly, some of whom you deeply know and love. Unfortunately, at times, they hurt you with their criticizing, manipulating, or intimidating words and actions. You may experience some of the same problems from people you don't know very well and, unfortunately, you may believe their hurtful words and give in to their unreasonable demands.

- Enjoying Skill #3 – "Counter a Negative with a Positive"
- Relating Skill #3 – "The C.A.L.M. Nice Guy Approach"
- Relating Skill #4 – "The C.U.T. Tough Guy Approach"
- Relating Skill #5 – "One Down Duck Down"
- Relating Skill #6 – "Disarm Them in the F.O.G."
- Relating Skill #7 – "Distracted Listening"

Pain Problem #7
"Underprepared for Pain Flares"

When pain flares come, you may feel unprepared to handle them and that adds to the hurt and upset. When you're caught off guard, you're likely to feel helpless and you might panic.

- Moving Skill #7 – "Flare Planning in Sets of Three"
- Moving Skill #8 – "Two Bottles of Comfort"

Pain Problem #8
"Missing the Good Things in Your Life"

Too often, pain and Misery dominate your attention so much that you may not notice the pleasures, positive changes, and other good events that are already happening inside and around you.

- Noticing Skill #3 – "I Want to See More of…"
- Noticing Skill #4 – "Comparison Questions"

Pain Problem #9 –
"Hypersensitive Nervous System"

Pain and stress have made your nervous system very sensitive to the pain signals traveling through it. In many cases, the brain has been altered by the ongoing pain and Misery experience, causing things that did not hurt in the past to hurt now. Also, what used to sting a little now stings a lot more (i.e., a pin prick feels like a knife cut)

- Re-Focusing Skill #1 – "Breath Count"
- Re-Focusing Skill #2 – "Breath Massage"
- Re-Focusing Skill #3 – "Mantra/Breath Meditation"
- Re-Focusing Skill #4 – "Mindfulness/Thought Labeling Meditation"
- Re-Focusing Skill #5 – "The Head Trip"
- Re-Focusing Skill #6 – "Self Hypnosis – Three Inductions"
- Re-Focusing Skills #7 – "Positive Distraction: The Fast and Slow Menus"
- Re-Focusing Skill #8 – "Immerse in a Good Memory"
- Enjoying Skill #1 – "Laughing"
- Enjoying Skill #2 – "Doing Fun"
- Enjoying Skill #3 – "Counter a Negative with a Positive"
- Enjoying Skill #4 – "Write a Gratitude Letter"
- Enjoying Skill #5 – "Filling a 'Good Stuff' Journal"

Pain Problem #10
"No Positive Future in Sight"

Too often, when chronic pain comes, he and Depression like to convince you that you no longer have a happy future. It's easy to believe this if you can no longer do your job or carry out everyday activities. You might feel like there is nothing good to look forward to.

- Moving Skill #1 – "Set a Goal, Create a Future"

Pain Problem #11
"Unbalanced Activity"

You find yourself drawn into activities that lead to pain flares, misery, and/or exhaustion. This often occurs when you over-do your activity (i.e., 3-hours of non-stop housecleaning), or under-do it (i.e., lying around a lot). This also happens if you engage in something that automatically flares the pain (i.e., lifting heavy objects).

- Moving Skill #2 – "Pay as You Go – Three Options"
- Moving Skill #3 – "The Payment Plan."

Pain Problem #12
"Poor Memory"

Your memory and concentration are compromised by many factors – pain, medication, low moods, anxiety, stress, and poor sleep.

- Re-Thinking Skill #1 – "Look in the Book"

Pain Problem #13
"Isolation and Loneliness"

You feel isolated and miserably alone, and/or you're terribly bored and this adds to your suffering and discomfort. This often occurs when you avoid good people or when the friends you thought you had abandon you.

- Relating Skill #1 – "Build New Relationships with Old Friends and Family"
- Relating Skill #2 – "How to Meet New Friends

Chapter Five – How to Use this Book - A Few Suggestions

Three Different Ways to Use this Book

I'm familiar with three groups of people who have their own approaches to reading and using self-help books:

- First, there are people who are **"Problem-Focused."** They manage things by taking action to solve particular difficulties first rather than learn an entire system of skills. If this is your style, turn to Chapter Five.

- A second group of people are **"Skill-Focused."** They feel more comfortable by learning and using a variety of methods, suggestions, and skills right away. If this is how you like to learn, start with Chapter Seven or Eight.

- Finally, there are individuals who are **"Learning-Focused."** They want to first review the background information about Problems and Skills before they jump into practicing. If this is how you like to learn, then go to "Appendix B," where you'll find a list of "Learn/Abouts." It shows you where you can find topics of interest that are spread throughout the book.

Many people may find that it is useful to draw from a mix of these approaches. Once you've completed the Introductions portion of the book, you may choose to use the Workbook in any way you'd like.

How to Use this Book – A Few More Suggestions

The next Info Box offers a few more suggestions as to how you might use this book. What's most important is that you make the program fit your needs.

INFO BOX #7
How to Use this Book –
A Few Suggestions

Suggestion #1 - Read through the Whole Book. If you prefer a thorough, detailed sense of what this approach offers, and the Skills it contains, read the entire book cover to cover.

Suggestion #2 – Start Small with the Brief Training Program. If you are ready to deal with a few Pain Problems and learn only one Comfort Skill to solve each, you can begin the Brief Training in Chapter Seven.

Suggestion #3 – Enter the Eight-Week Basic Training Program. If you want a more comprehensive training, and you are ready to make a larger time commitment, skip over to Chapter Eight, and take the course. *Remember* that even though this longer Training is presented as a set of interconnected lesson plans, you can do it at your own pace. For example, you may decide to spend a month or more working on one week's worth of Skills.

Suggestion #4 – Focus on Your Own Mix of Skills. If you want to pick a particular Comfort Skill, draw from the collection listed in "Appendix A". You can put together a selection of these and make your own training program, one that will move you towards your own Comfort goals

Suggestion #5 - Do It Any Way You Want. Maybe you have your own ideas as to how you want to use this book. Go for it!

Free Online Resource – Relaxation Recording

In addition to reading the various Learning Options, when you can, log onto ComfortClinic.org and take advantage of a number of free resources provided there, including a free-access relaxation recording led by the author.

Your Notes

The Comfort Skills Workbook

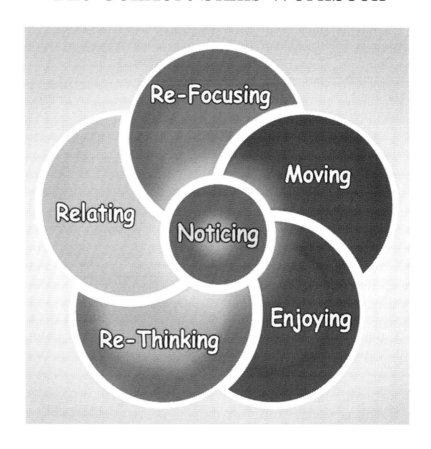

Chapter Six – Workbook Introduction

This Workbook provides you two learning options. Both will train you in a number of Comfort Skills that you can use to solve the Pain Problems that make you miserable and worsen chronic pain.

The first learning option is **"Problem-Focused"** and lists thirteen Pain Problems and the Comfort Skills that Solve Them. People who want to focus their energies on solving a particular difficulty will find Chapter Four useful in locating the Comfort Skills that will help them solve a particular problem.

The second learning option is **"Skill-Focused"** and guides the reader in acquiring the general techniques and methods that have helped people-in-pain to reduce Misery and pain. It offers two trainings:

- In Chapter Seven, **"The Brief Training,"** you'll find a detailed description of six Pain Problems that correspond to the six Comfort Strategies. Instructions on how to use the corresponding Skill are also included. The chapter also offers an additional, "Bonus" Problem and Skill, which brings the total to seven. This chapter also reviews background information on some of the problems and Skills.

- The **"Eight-Week Basic Training"** in Chapter Eight is more comprehensive than the Brief Training. It includes thirty-six Comfort Skills that you can learn over an eight-week period or longer. These will help you to solve the thirteen Pain Problems described in Chapter Six.

Chapter Seven – The Brief Training

Brief Training Contents Box

Introduction to the Brief Training
1. Seven Pain Problems
2. Brief Training and Format

Solving Pain Problem #1
"Unpredictable Pain Flares and Emotional Distress"
1. Solve it with the Noticing Strategy
2. Learn/About Negatives – "Triggers" and "First Signs"
3. Do It Now!
   A) *Noticing Skill #1 – "Revealing Triggers"*
4. Homework Box

Solving Pain Problem #2
"Attention Hijacked by Pain and Stress"
1. Solve it with the Re-Focusing Strategy
2. Do It Now!
   A) *Re-Focusing Skill #1 - "Breath Count"*
4. Homework Box

Solving Pain Problem #3
"Poor Sleep and Rest at Night"
1. Solve it with the Moving Strategy
2. Learn/About Sleep and Rest
3. Do It Now!
   A) *Moving Skill #5 – "Rest in the Bed"*
4. Homework Box

Solving Pain Problem #4
"Sadness, Worry and Other Miserable Feelings"

1. Solve it with the Enjoying Strategy
2. Learn/About Positive Psychology
3. Do It Now!
   A) *Enjoying Skill #2 – "Doing Fun"*
4. Homework Box

Solving Pain Problem #5
"Negative Thoughts"

1. Solve it with the Re-Thinking Strategy
2. Learn/About Negative Thoughts
3. Do It Now!
   A) *Re-Thinking Skill #2 – "See It Coming"*
4. Homework Box

Solving Pain Problem #6
"Distress Caused by Annoying People"

1. Solve it with the Relating Strategy
2. Learn/About Annoying People, Toxic Talk, and Saying "No!
3. Do It Now!
   A) *Relating Skill #1 – "The C.A.L.M., Nice Guy Approach"*
4. Homework Box

BONUS
Solving Pain Problem #7
"Underprepared for Pain Flares"

1. Solve it with the Moving Strategy - Pain Flare Planning
2. Do It Now!
   A) *Moving Skill #7 – "Flare Planning in Sets of Three"*
3. Homework Box

Introduction to the Brief-Training

Pain Problems

In this Training, you will learn about seven Pain Problems and how to use a Comfort Skill to solve each one.

INFO BOX #9 –
Seven Sample Pain Problems

1. Unpredictable Pain Flares and Emotional Distress

2. Attention Hijacked by Pain and Stress

3. Poor Sleep and Rest at Night

4. Sadness, Worry, and Other Miserable Feelings

5. Negative Thoughts

6. Distress Caused by Annoying People

7. Underprepared for Pain Flares

Brief-Training Format

If you recall from Chapter One, I organize the Comfort Skills into six categories called "Comfort Strategies." These Strategies include Noticing, Re-Focusing, Moving, Enjoying, Re-Thinking, and Relating.[26] You may think of this Brief Training as a sampling of one Comfort Skill from each of the Strategies. I'll also add one more as a "Bonus," giving you seven. Each of the sections follow the format displayed in the nest Box:

INFO BOX #10 –
Brief-Training Format

The Pain Problem. Each of the seven sections in this Brief Training will begin with a common difficulty that you face as a person-in-pain.

Solve it with the _____ Strategy. This highlights one of the six Comfort Strategies included in the training and briefly describes the Strategy and the Skills it contains.

---

[26] They are visually depicted on a "Comfort Wheel;" find it in Chapter One.

Learn/About _____ . This provides addition information about a particular Pain Problem, Strategy, or Skill.

Do it Now! Here you are given the specific instructions you'll need to practice the relevant Comfort Skill. You're also encouraged to practice that Skill soon after you learn about it.

Homework Box. As the saying goes, "Repetition is the mother of learning." You'll find it very useful to practice the Skill several times before moving on to the next section.

Remember

- **Take Your Time**. Some of you may give yourself a week or more to work on one Pain Problem. Others of you might want to do more. No matter how you choose to learn, make sure that it is done at a comfortable pace.

The Journal

A number of Skill Boxes will instruct you to do some writing. You may find it very useful to buy a blank journal and turn it into your "Brief Training" or "Comfort Skill" Journal. You can keep a number of notes and other writings in that one book and review them from time to time.

Solving Pain Problem #1 – "Unpredictable Pain Flares and Emotional Distress"

The Problem: Difficulties like pain flares and emotional upsets seem to come out of nowhere, leaving you feeling helpless and frustrated.

Solve it with the Noticing Strategy

The first of the six Strategies on the Comfort Wheel includes the **"Noticing Strategy**," *which is the practice of making yourself aware of the positive and negative events that occur in your daily life.* The expression "to notice" derives from the Greek *"Noscere"* meaning to "come to know." When you direct your awareness towards a situation, you are in a better position to understand and describe it. When you don't use your ability to notice, you'll have little or no idea about what you're dealing with.

The Noticing Strategy includes four Skills (two of which are described below). The first two Skills help you notice the "Negatives" that warn you when a pain flare or emotional upset is coming. ***In order to solve a problem, it's often necessary to first recognize it***, then it becomes easier to use other Comfort Skills to reduce the size and influence of pain flares and emotional distress.

The last two Noticing Skills focus you on some of the "Positives" that come your way. Often, chronic pain and low moods obscure your perception and you can't see anything positive happening. However, as you use the Positive Noticing Skills, you'll become happily surprised to discover that Positives have been there all along. And, as you notice them, they tend to increase, especially if you are using other Comfort Skills or your own resources. (You'll find Positive Noticing Skills listed in the "Basic Training" course in Chapter Eight.)

Learn/About Negatives – "Triggers" and "First Signs"

A **Negative** *is an event that either sets off or warns you that a pain flare, stress, or emotional upset is on the way .* Two types are "Triggers" and "First Signs."

1. **Triggers** *are events or situations that set off bad moods, stress, and pain flares.* (i.e., bright lights often set off Migraine headaches, or criticism can enrage a person). Triggers often originate outside of you in the physical or social world. Sometimes activities or habits can act like a Trigger.

2. **First Signs** *are your responses to a Trigger – these warn you that you are heading for a pain flare, stress, or emotional upset.* You'll sometimes notice it happening in your body, emotions, mind, and/or in behavior, which might include muscle tension, hopeless thoughts, depressing images, or over-eating.

Chicken or the Egg? – An Example

Some of you might find it difficult to tell the difference between a "Trigger" and a "First Sign." It may not always be necessary to do this. Here is one example to illustrate the differences: Let's say that you have a low-back injury, and you bend over one time to pick up something – that is an Activity Trigger. Fairly soon, you notice that your back muscles begin to tense up a little – that sensation is a First Sign. If you don't avoid the Trigger (bending and lifting) or you don't listen to the warning of that First Sign (muscle ache) you might bend over and lift something several times and eventually suffer from a major pain flare. In the end, it doesn't matter whether or not you define and act on something happening as a Trigger or a First Sign – as long as you notice the Negatives that come before a pain flare or upsetting emotion, you'll be able to 1) predict when a problem is coming, and 2) do something to change it. The next Info Box describes these Negatives.

INFO BOX #11 –
Negative Triggers and First Signs

Triggers. These tend to cause physical or emotional distress, which increases pain. Three broad categories include the following:

- *Physical Triggers.* Things you see or feel in your physical surroundings that cause problems. Examples – bad weather, loud noises.
- *Social Triggers.* People in your life who irritate you and worsen pain and stress. Examples – A nagging spouse or annoying co-worker.
- *Activity Triggers.* There are things you do that can set off episodes of discomfort. Examples – Lifting heavy weight or lying around a lot.

First Signs. These happen to your body and mind when you're exposed to a Trigger. First Signs warn you that a pain flare or distressing event is coming. There are five different types:

- *Physical First Signs*. Many come in the form of body sensations such as tight neck/shoulders, a rapid heartbeat, sudden fatigue, or achy feet.
- *Thought First Signs*. In reaction to a Trigger, your mind often turns to negative thoughts (i.e., When asking for help you might think: "I'm a burden on everyone").
- *Imagined First Signs*. What you see, hear, and feel in your imagination can alert you that pain and distress are coming (i.e., imagining an argument you once had with someone).
- *Emotional First Signs*. Feelings such as anxiety, anger, and sadness warn you that you've become vulnerable to a flare.
- *Behavioral First Signs*. Some of your actions may indicate that a problem is imminent (i.e., rushing around nervously, yelling at people).

STORY BOX #2 –
The Negatives of Chocolate Cake

Thirty-five-year-old Jane suffered from damaged knees. After learning that each pound of her body weight put four pounds of pressure on her knees, she decided to go on a diet. She thought that if she could lose some weight, she'd get some relief. For five months, she'd been trying to meet her goals, but found that this was very difficult. One challenging moment came along one day when she felt a gnawing hunger in the pit of her stomach. The problem was that this happened right after she finished lunch! In addition to this, she also experienced thoughts that said things like, "Oh boy, a hot fudge sundae would be a great end to lunch," and "That Danish I had on Saturday was really delicious." She was also a little upset because in the morning she had a big argument with her mother on the phone. This caused her to replay angry thoughts in her head again and again, such as, "My mother is so unfair." She decided to do some housework to forget the call and she ended up doing too much, causing a moderate pain flare in her knees.

As if this wasn't bad enough, when she hobbled into the living room, she found a chocolate cake in an open bakery box sitting on the coffee table. Apparently, her husband brought a treat home for the kids. Jane looked at it for a long time and, as she tried to walk away, a sudden image flashed in her mind. She saw herself seated at the kitchen table with a glass of milk and a large chunk of chocolate cake. That was it! – she turned around and turned her fantasy into a reality by eating the cake. Suffice it to say that she didn't lose weight that day.

Unlike the painful situation that you are going through, Jane was focusing on how her Triggers and First Signs alerted her about the urges of sugar-eating. The next Box uses Jane's story to help you identify the Triggers and First Signs that caused her difficulties.

INFO BOX #12 –
The Negatives in Jane's Story

Jane's Triggers. These pushed her to eat fattening foods.

- *Physical Trigger.* The chocolate cake sitting on the living room table.
- *Social Trigger.* The criticizing tone and words from her mother that she heard on the phone (which stressed her out).
- *Activity Trigger.* She did too much housework and that created pain. This added discomfort made her vulnerable to use something familiar to soothe herself (i.e., the cake).

Jane's First Signs. All of the signs described below warned Jane that the urge to eat sweets was on its way.

- *Physical First Signs.* She felt muscle tension in her shoulders after arguing with her mother. This caused her to seek relief from physical stress (i.e., by doing comfort-eating).
- *Thought First Signs.* Jane angrily thought "my mother is so unfair!" and "A hot fudge sundae would taste good now." The first thought motivated her to seek something to calm herself and the second gave her the bad idea of what that could be.
- *Imagined First Signs.* She imagined herself feeling better while eating chocolate cake. This is a very "dangerous" image for a person trying to diet.
- *Emotional First Signs.* Jane felt a rush of upsetting emotions that were set off by the phone call with her mother. These included feelings of anger, guilt, and sadness. These feelings (a) motivated her to seek something fast to soothe her and, (b) drew her to an unhealthy choice.
- *Behavioral First Signs.* As she walked through the living room, she stopped and looked at the cake for a long time. She also took steps towards it and eventually picked it up.

After looking over the following two Info Boxes, you can start your training by using the following Skill Boxes. These will train you in how to identify Triggers.

INFO BOX #13 -
Sample Triggers that Increase Pain Flares

- Obsessing on Anxious Thoughts
- Lack of Sleep
- Focusing on Bad Memories or the Pain
- Imagining a Painful Future
- Impatient Feelings
- Multi-Tasking
- Annoying People
- Unhealthy Foods
- Intense Stimulation (i.e., Loud Noises)
- Extreme Work or Activity Load
- Arguments

INFO BOX #14 -
Sample First Signs that Warn You About Pain Flares

- Confusion, Overwhelm and Sadness
- Worry and Anxiety
- Muscle Tension
- Fast Heart Beats
- Boredom
- Sleeplessness and Fatigue
- Feelings of Hopelessness and Helplessness
- Loneliness

Do It Now!

Noticing Skill #1 – "Revealing Triggers"

This Skill Box describes one method you can use to identify a Trigger.

NOTICING SKILL BOX #1 -
"Revealing Triggers"

Step One- Revealing Triggers. After a pain flare passes, think back to what was going on the previous day or two before the flare hit you. Identify the Triggers in your Physical, Social, and Activity Worlds that may have set it off. Here are some useful questions:

A) *Physical Triggers.* Ask yourself:
- "What was the weather like?"
- "Did I have a cold, flu, or other illness?"
- "Were there loud sounds or intense smells that irritated me?"

B) *Social Triggers.* Ask yourself:
- "Did anyone annoy me before the flare?"
- "Did I hear some bad news regarding someone I care about?"
- "Did a friend or family member just criticize me?"

C) *Activity Triggers.* Ask yourself:
- "What activities did I do before the flare came?"
- "How many strenuous activities did I do?"
- "Did I get stressed out while doing something today?"

D) *Other Triggers.* "Did I get an unexpected bill on the mail?"

Step Two - Make a Trigger List. Using a journal or digital file, record the Triggers that you identified.

Step Three - Watch Out for "Repeaters." Once you've made your list, notice any Triggers that happen a lot. Each time you notice this, pull out your list and place a check mark after this repeating Trigger. This Step can better help you to catch and disarm that Trigger.

Step Four - Add to the List. Over the weeks and months, add to the List new Triggers and Repeaters that you discover. If you'd like, keep a copy with you.

Step Five – Using Your Trigger List. The list will alert you to the Triggers that pop up and remind you to disarm them by using some of the other Comfort Skills. In this way, you can better control your relationship with pain. For example, if arguing with your spouse is a Trigger, you can 1) stop the argument, 2) use the "Breath Count" Skill to calm your nervous system, and 3) do something fun to raise your mood.

NOTICING HOMEWORK BOX

1. **Revealing Triggers.** Using the Noticing Skill above to identify Triggers that set off flares and/or upsetting situations. Write some of these down in your Journal.

Solving Pain Problem #2 – "Attention Hijacked by Pain and Stress"

The Problem: Your attention becomes overly absorbed by pain as well as stress, anxiety, and/or other emotional upsets. This is because you have unknowingly allowed yourself to focus on these difficulties and your brain has grown used to directing its attention towards them.

Solve it with the Re-Focusing Strategy

Attention can very powerfully influence pain and Comfort. Here is an analogy: Like many teenagers, when I was a kid, I used to love squirting a stream of lighter fluid onto a campfire and watching the flames shoot up. Imagine that pain is like a fire, and your attention is like a stream of lighter fluid – if you aim a stream of fluid at the fire…well, you get the idea. When you combine pain-focusing with helpless, hopeless, and other catastrophic thoughts and feelings, you get a lot more pain and Misery.[27] The good news is that you can learn how to re-direct your attention towards Comfort.

"Re-Focusing Strategy" *is a set of Skills that direct your attention towards something neutral or pleasant*.[28] The regular practice of these Skills helps you to build up your "concentration muscle." This enables you to take back your attention from pain and stress. As you use Re-Focusing Skills, you'll be in a better position to soothe and desensitize your nervous system, relax your mind and body, and reduce pain and emotional distress. These techniques can also potentially lower blood pressure, decrease tension, enhance immunity to disease, reduce depression and anxiety, and increase pain relief and tolerance. Re-Focusing Skills include Positive Distraction, Breathing practices, Meditation, Imagery, and Self-Hypnosis.

---

[27] Google "Reconceptualising Pain According to Modern Pain Science," by G. Lorimer Moseley.
[28] This book uses the term "Re-Focusing" as defined above. It is no way related to the "Refocusing" method developed by the spiritual direction counselor, Dr. Diane Divett, or to the "Refocus Step" created by Dr Jeffrey Schwartz, or to any other method.

Re-Focusing Skills – Two Actions that Change Your Body

Most Re-Focusing Skills include two actions. When you engage in them, they create calming and pleasant changes in your body and mind. They also help you to move away from irritating distractions such as pain, loud sounds, and negative thoughts.

- **Action One – "Let Go and Relax."** The first thing to do is relax your mind and body as best you can. Allow your muscles to soften and let thoughts, feelings, sounds, or other distractions come and go without dwelling on or fighting them. Just let them be there and take on a "laid back attitude." Do your best to chill out and take it easy. In this way, you'll release the distractions and prevent yourself from trying too hard to <u>make</u> something happen. When you notice that you are distracted by something, just let it go and gently return to focus. Allow the Comfort to come in its own time.

- **Action Two – "Focus on One Thing."** As you "Let Go and Relax," you also "Focus on One Thing" by aiming your attention, like a laser beam, at something pleasant or neutral. Keep your focus there. You might concentrate on your breath, on the sound of water, on a happy memory, or even on a good word repeated over and over in your mind.

By putting these two core actions together, Let Go and Relax and Focus on One Thing, your body will eventually learn how to fill with comfortable and relaxing sensations.[29] The Skills in this Strategy will include these two Actions. We'll first begin with the "Breath Count."

Re-Focusing Practice Tips

The best way for your brain to benefit from Re-Focusing Skills is to practice them while you are alert. You may encounter several obstacles as you use the Re-Focusing Skills – one is unintended sleep. As you practice the "Breath Count," for example, it may relax you to the point that you'll fall into a deep sleep. What causes you to fall asleep during this exercise is your brain – it has learned over many years that when you sit or lie still, close your eyes, and allow your mind to rest…. It's bed time! It will take some weeks and months of practice before your brain learns that you are not trying to go to sleep, but, instead, you are entering into a place of Comfort.

---

[29] When you practice them, your body shifts into a state called the "Relaxation Response." See the book: "The Relaxation Response," by Herbert Benson.

RE-FOCUSING SKILL TIPS BOX

1. **Awake Seating.** Choose a seating arrangement that comfortably fits your body. However, in order to move in and out of a relaxed state without falling asleep, select a chair or recliner that's comfortable but won't easily put you to sleep. (If you want to use the Skill to help you sleep and rest, practice in bed at night.)

2. **Avoid the "Lie-Down."** Until your brain has learned the difference between going into a relaxed Comfort state and sleep, its best to avoid practicing the Skill while lying down (but OK to do at bedtime).

3. **Choose Calm, Quiet Surroundings.** When you're starting out, it's good to practice in a place that is quiet and has few distractions (i.e., away from kids, telephones, loud people). *Calm Car:* If this is difficult to find in your home, use your car as a quiet practice space. Some people drive to a peaceful spot nearby, park, lock their doors, and practice the Re-Focusing Skill while sitting in the car. As you gain more experience with the Skill, you'll be able to calmly focus at home even in the presence of distracting noises.

4. **"Just Do It to Do It."** The more you use a Re-Focusing Skill, the more often you'll encounter a sense of calm throughout your whole body. One problem you may come across is that, after having a good experience with it, you expect the same thing to happen each time you practice the Skill. This expectation may pressure you to try too hard and doing that produces more stress than Comfort. It's best to "just do it to do it" and <u>replace desperate trying and seeking with calm, curious noticing</u>. Just observe what happens and *allow the Comfort to come in its own time.*

5. **Tracking Practice Time.** Like most people, you probably want to know when your practice session is over so that you can move on to other things. In order to do that, and not have to open your eyes to look at your watch, use one of these methods to keep track of the time:
   A) Set a timer.
   B) Use a recording that guides you in a Re-Focusing Skill; when the track is over, you're done.
   C) Use a set of *Meditation Beads* (see page 228).

> 6. **WARNING!!** – Occasionally, while practicing some Re-Focusing Skills (i.e., the Breath Count), you may perceive a little increase in pain. This is because you are Re-Focusing your attention away from some of the things in your daily life that distract you from pain (i.e., conversations with people, eating, taking a walk). This is also part of the reason why you feel more discomfort at night – while in bed, you are not distracted by your usual activities. If pain happens to rise during a Re-Focusing exercise, you'll find it helpful to do one of the following: **a)** stop practicing that Skill at that moment and try it later, **b)** change the Re-Focusing Skill you use (i.e., from Breathing to Imagery), or **c)** consider the pain as a distraction, let it be there, relax around it, and return to focus (this can eventually result in more Comfort).

Do It Now!

Re-Focusing Skill #1 – "Breath Count"

We breathe all of the time. ("How good is that!?) The **"Breath Count"** Skill is a relatively easy one to use because breathing is a natural function of your body – the wonderful and convenient thing about your breath is that you carry it with you wherever you go, making it easy to use as you change your physiology and generate relief and calm. When you practice the "Breath Count," you may feel like you're counting sheep without the sheep. It comes from the Zen Meditation tradition and combines two forms of concentration: **1) Physical Concentration** (Re-Focusing on the feeling of your breath moving in and out of your belly or chest), and **2) Mental Concentration** (counting numbers silently in your mind). Scientists have demonstrated that the "Breath Count" and other forms of Meditation powerfully help you redirect your attention away from pain and towards more calm and Comfort.[30]

---

[30] "Full Catastrophe Living: Using the wisdom of the Body and the Mind to Face Stress, Pain, and Illness" by Jon Kabat-Zinn, Ph.D.

RE-FOCUSING SKILL BOX #1 –
"The Breath Count"

Step One - Quiet Place and Timer. First, find a quiet place to sit and set a timer for five (or more) minutes. Choose a seat or recliner that supports your body. Remember, if you lie down, you may fall asleep.

Step Two - Breaths in the Belly. Start with a couple of deep breaths and focus on the feeling of your belly moving in and out. Then, continue following your natural breath. If the belly is an uncomfortable place to focus on, choose another part of your body (i.e., hands), and imagine the breath moving in and out of there.

Step Three - Breath Count. As you breathe naturally, count each exhale quietly in your mind. After ten breaths, start again at one. If you lose count, simply start with the number one. Variation – as you inhale, think the word "and" (i.e., inhale - "and," exhale - "one"). Continue counting each cycle of ten until your practice time is up.

Step Four - Returning. After the timer goes off, take three slow, deep breaths and as you exhale for the third time, allow your eyes to slowly open. Take time to "awaken" from the experience; walk around a little.

Remember - Let Distractions Be There and Re-Focus
When a distracting thought, memory, image, feeling, sound, or anything tries to move your mind away from the breath, let it be there and return your mind back to focus. Don't fight the distractions; simply re-focus your attention back to the breath and the count.

Okay, now use the Skill Box above to sit for at least five-to-ten minutes and practice the "Breath Count."

RE-FOCUSING HOMEWORK BOX

1. **Re-Focusing at Home.** Practice the "Breath Count" for 10 to 20 minutes each day (see Skill Box above).

2. **"Extra Credit" – Triggers and Re-Focusing Skills.** Identify Triggers that set off flares and/or upsetting situations. When you notice these coming your way, use the "Breath Count" for 10 to 20 minutes to help you prevent or reduce the stress that this Trigger causes. (See page 81.)

Solving Pain Problem #3 – "Poor Sleep and Rest at Night"

The Problem: You feel exhausted and achy in the morning because you had a difficult time falling and/or staying asleep. In part, this is because you may be dealing with many distractions, physical and psychological, that keep you awake.

Solve it with the Moving Strategy

The **"Moving Strategy"** *is the practice of moving comfortably and confidently through four tasks which are common to people-in-pain: Goal Setting, Moving the Body, Sleep and Rest, and Pain Flare Planning.* The following expands upon these:

1. **Goal Setting**. Too often, Pain and Depression tell you that "you have no future." This Skill shows you how to counter that lie by offering you a way to develop personal goals and pursue a new future. Each goal you work on brings you closer to a new, meaningful future.
2. **Moving the Body.** This skill-set helps you to find balance in your physical activity and reduce pain flares related to over- or under-doing activity.
3. **Sleep and Rest.** You may ask yourself, "How can I get more sleep and rest?" Granted, sleep has become very difficult for most of you since pain and other distractions disturb you at night. Sleep Skills will improve your bedtime rest.
4. **Pain Flare Planning**. These Skills help you to move more comfortably through pain flares.

Learn/About Sleep and Rest

"To rise in the morning like a roaring lion,
you need to lie down at night like a quiet lamb."
Proverb

In my workshops, I often ask everyone, "Who sleeps fairly well at night?" At most, one or two folks raise their hands. I know that most of you have a terrible time falling and staying asleep. I also know that it's not necessary to quote all of the scientific and health literature to convince you that losing sleep causes Misery and increased pain the next day. In the following sections we'll look at how sleep and rest work, and how you can get more out of them.

89

How Sleep Works

What controls your body's ability to get restful sleep? It's the brain, of course. The scientific name for one brain process that influences the quantity and quality of your sleep is the "Circadian Rhythm." The more stable and consistent your Circadian Rhythm functions, the better you sleep.

Your Internal Clock

One way to understand this is to imagine that you have an "Internal Clock" located in the middle of your head.[31] When it's working well, it will ease you into sleep and raise you up refreshed and energetic in the morning. Many of you might recall that, in the past, you could wake up before the alarm clock went off in the morning and also feel very sleepy about the same time at night. For the most part, your Internal Clock was working pretty well.

Sleep and Chronic Pain

Although you may have slept fairly well in the past, chronic pain has now come along and is challenging your nights. The sleep-time many of you used to have is now interrupted by pain, depression, stress, and worry. A collection of scientific studies over the last two decades show that pain and low moods interfere with important sleep states and leave you exhausted in the morning.[32] What's worse, when you're deprived of sleep, pain flares increase in intensity and frequency and that can disturb your sleep even more.[33]

Re-Setting Your Clock

So how do pain, depression, worry, medications, and poor sleep habits interfere with your night-time slumber? The answer is that they "throw your clock off." Sleep is a very sensitive brain function regulated by your Internal Clock. There are a whole host of sleep Skills that help you to re-set that clock and return you to a better level of sleep and rest. One of three such Skills is described next.

---

[31] For more information, you can read "The Promise of Sleep," by Dr William C. Dement.

[33] Lautenbacher, S, Kundermann, B, & Krieg, J.C. (2006). Sleep deprivation and pain perception, Sleep Medicine Review, Volume 10(#5): Pages 357-369; Roehrs, T, & Roth, T (2005). Sleep and pain: interaction of two vital functions, Seminars in Neurology, Volume 25(#1): Pages 106-116

Do It Now!

Changing the Bed of Sleeplessness

A good number of you who have trouble falling or staying asleep at night may lie awake for a long while and toss and turn in bed! After a while, you might decide to get up and do things like watch TV, eat, "surf the Net," or play video games. These activities may exhaust you to the point that you'll return to bed and collapse into a deep sleep (or you may "conk out" in a chair in the living room). An hour or two later, you might wake up and the whole process will start all over again!

Many of you are unaware that you have unintentionally transformed your bed into a "Tossing and Turning Station." When you lie awake in bed longer than 15-20 minutes, you're accidentally teaching your brain that the bed is for tossing and turning. Because your bed is not a peaceful resting spot, it may be difficult for you to ease down into a pleasant slumber. In the next story, Meenah found a creative way to teach her brain to transform her bed into a place of rest and relaxation.

STORY BOX #3 – Meenah Changes Beds

Meenah is a 24-year-old nurse who gets migraine headaches. She told me that one night she found herself tossing and turning and couldn't get to sleep, even after getting up and down out of bed a couple of times. One night, she came up with an idea – she would switch her sleeping position by putting her head where her feet were. Within five minutes, she was out! Apparently, her brain perceived this new position as a "different bed," one that she could sleep in. This helped her to overcome the thoughts and feelings that kept her awake.

Moving Skill #7 – "Rest in the Bed"

This Skill is one way to calm the restlessness you feel in bed at night. It's based on studies that compared meditators and sleepers. In one experiment, researchers observed two groups of people, one that slept for eight hours and the other that meditated for two 20-minute sessions each day. The scientists looked at the brain waves each group emitted and found that the meditators' brains entered a sleep state similar to that of the eight-hour sleepers. Even better, the meditative brains registered the same amount of time in "Delta," which is a slow brain-wave associated with a good night's sleep. [34]

---

[34] See the 1977 article in the journal, Psychophysiology entitled "Physiological changes in Yoga meditation," by B.D. Elson and colleagues, Volume 14, number 1, pages 55-57; the 1976 article in Science, "Sleep during

This is great news! If you can't sleep you have another option: You can rest by practicing any Re-Focusing Skill in bed ALL NIGHT LONG. Many of my workshop attendees used one or more Skills, drawing from Breathing Techniques, Imagery, Meditation, and Self-Hypnosis (all found in the Basic Training Program, Chapter Eight). When they did this, they either 1) fell asleep, or 2) comfortably rested throughout the night. In the morning, they all felt more rested and energized. The next Skill Box describes how you can do this.

MOVING SKILL BOX #5 -
"Rest in the Bed"

Step One – Give Up Sleep and Take a Rest. After 20 minutes awake in bed, give up sleep. Do not try to go to sleep that night; just rest.

Step Two – Turn Clock Around. If you are in the habit of looking at your bedside clock at night, you may have noticed that doing that will add to your stress and keep you awake. Free yourself from this by turning the clock around so you can't see its face.

Step Three – Rest in the Bed. Allow yourself to rest all night long by practicing the "Breath Count" and/or other Re-Focusing Skills (see page 338 for a list of these Skills). If you fall asleep and wake up later in the night, repeat these Steps if you can't get back to sleep in twenty minutes.

Remember
- **"Replace Desperate Trying with Calm Noticing."** Be careful to avoid trying to go to sleep. "Trying" rarely works because most of us try too hard – and when we do we end up anxiously looking for a change. If good results don't happen immediately, we get upset, discouraged, and give up - or we try harder and become even more frustrated. Instead:
  - ➤ "Just do it to do it," and
  - ➤ Curiously notice what happens, instead of desperately trying to make things happen. Allow good results to come in their own time.

- **Adjust Yourself.** Feel free to adjust your body for Comfort as much as you want throughout the night, then refocus on the Skill practice.

Transcendental Meditation, " by R.R. Pagano and L.R. Frumkin, Volume 191, pages 308-309; the 1975 article in Perceptual and Motor Skills, Sleep during Transcendental Meditation, " by J. Younger and colleagues, Volume 40, number 3, pages 953-954.

"MOVING" HOMEWORK BOX

1. **Breath Counting at Home.** Practice the "Breath Count" for 10 to 20 minutes each day.

2. **Notice Triggers to Remind You to Practice.** When you notice a stressful Trigger (i.e., annoying person criticizing you) draw on one of the Comfort Skills above (i.e., go to a quiet place and practice the "Breath Count").

3. **"Resting in Bed."** Using this Moving Skill to improve your night-time rest and sleep.

Solving Pain Problem #4 –
"Sadness, Worry, and Other Miserable Feelings"

The Problem: You find little pleasure in life and often feel depressed, angry, worried, and/or bored. These feelings are often brought on by the uncomfortable sensations you feel in your body. These miseries are making it difficult for you to feel pleasure or anything good.

Solve it with the Enjoying Strategy

Enjoying Strategy is the practice of raising your mood, positively coping with upsetting situations, and strengthening your positive qualities and sense of personal meaning. Enjoying helps you diminish discomfort and sadness and, instead, pursue healthy pleasures and happy moments.

Sounds too simple, right?! That's because for most of you, it's difficult to do pleasurable things when you're hurting or feeling depressed, anxious or angry. It makes sense that when you're feeling bad, advice such as "Follow Your Bliss" or "Don't Worry, Be Happy" sounds like namby-pamby, FuFu, self-help kaka! So, it might surprise you to learn that when you engage in joyful activities and cultivate positive thoughts and attitudes, you will eventually experience a good feeling that grows and expands. This has been established by years of research.[35] As you raise your mood, you become more creative, productive, healthy, and, most importantly, more comfortable. Enjoying Skills are divided into three categories: 1) "Enjoying Right Now," 2) "Making a Positive U-Turn" away from a challenging moment, and 3) "Cultivating Positive Qualities" that create a life of lasting happiness and personal meaning.

Learn/About Positive Psychology

Recent discoveries about the power of positive emotions come from the work of many researchers in a relatively new field. **Positive Psychology *is the scientific study, and practical application, of the positive strengths that enable individuals and communities to thrive*.**[36] Up until the late 1990s, most traditional research and practice in psychology focused on the problems that happen in the mind and brain. This approach was borrowed from the medical world and is called the "Disease Model." Healthcare providers and scientists who follow this orientation are primarily interested in studying conditions such as depression, panic attacks, substance abuse, and chronic pain. These professionals are

---

[35] "The How of Happiness: A New Approach to Getting the Life You Want" by Sonja Lyubomirsky, Ph.D., and "A Primer in Positive Psychology" by Christopher Peterson.
[36] Adapted from the Positive Psychology Center website.

interested in developing treatments that directly cure or change these problems. Using this approach, practitioners of Behavioral, Psychodynamic, and especially Cognitive-Behavioral therapies have helped people reduce their physical and psychological suffering.

In 1998, a group of psychologists, headed by Dr. Martin Seligman, banded together and decided to study "happy people." They observed that the field of psychology was shaped by the study of sad and miserable people and was not focusing enough attention on individuals who were joyful and living a productive, contented life. The group of psychologists who decided to study these people called their collective efforts the "Positive Psychology Movement." It promotes the idea that "…human goodness and excellence are as authentic as disease, disorder, and distress."[37] They investigated the resilience, self-empowerment, and positive values that happy people applied to difficult situations. Investigators also looked at what made people happy and able to overcome life's obstacles and challenges. They asked, "What kind of positive attitudes and behaviors do these folks have and how do their personal qualities impact their mental and physical health?" From their findings, some of these scientists created Positive Psychology exercises that empower people to increase joy and personal satisfaction. [38]

I include some of these exercises, along with other positive practices, in the Enjoying Strategy because positive mood is intimately connected to your health and well-being. In other words, when you do things to increase your happiness and positive feelings, and you strengthen your positive qualities, you're better able to enhance your Comfort.

Do It Now!

Enjoying Skill #2 – "Doing Fun"

For many of you, life doesn't feel as fun as it was in the past. Some of you have given up on seeking the things that once gave you pleasure. True, there are activities that you can no longer do comfortably, but there are plenty of new ones out there waiting for you. You might also find that you're able to return to old pleasures by doing them a different way (i.e, walking fifteen minutes in a park instead of trekking five miles up a mountain trail). Like other Skills, when you practice "Doing Fun," it's like building a muscle – the more you exercise it, the stronger you get. The following Skill Box offers one way to return to Fun.

---

[37] "A Primer in Positive Psychology," by Christopher Peterson.
[38] "The How of Happiness" by Sonja Lyubomirsky and "Learned Optimism" by Martin Seligman.

ENYOYING SKILL BOX #2 -
"Doing Fun"

Brain Storm and Experiment. Here is one way to discover the activities you'll enjoy doing:

- *Step One - Get Ready.* Sit down comfortably with pen and paper, or with a journal or digital file.
- *Step Two - Recall.* Close your eyes, let your mind roam through your memory and recall:
    i.   What you used to enjoy doing
    ii. What you think you might enjoy doing
    iii. What enjoyable things you've been doing lately
    iv. What you haven't done but are interested in trying
- *Step Three – Write the List.* Write these down and don't edit them.
- *Step Four – Order the List.* Next, order the items on the list from those activities you want to do right away to those that can wait.
- *Step Five - Choose It and Do It.* Pick an activity from the list and decide how you'll carry it out -- Then, do it!
- *Step Six - Evaluate.* Soon after you finish the activity, think about it. Did you have fun? What worked; what didn't? Would you like to do it again, modify it, or put it away?
- *Step Seven - Do Another One.* Repeat Steps Five and Six as many times as you'd like.

The Fun Menus. Once you've identified and/or tried out several enjoyable things to do, you can create a couple of "menus" that include some of your favorite activities.

A) *The "Quick Fun Menu."* This is made up of activities you can begin doing within an hour or so. Example – Perhaps you'll decide to go to a café and read a book, go for a walk, call a friend, watch a movie or a ball game on TV, or eat a nice meal at a local restaurant.

B) *The "Big Fun Menu."* This Menu has activities that'll take some time to prepare for and carry out, and they're well worth it. Example – Perhaps taking a short trip with a friend or a sweetheart to a Bed-and-Breakfast hotel for a weekend, or attending a music festival.

BONUS. Lean how to Do Fun (and other activities) differently on page 164.

ENJOYING HOMEWORK BOX

1. **Breath Counting.** Practice the "Breath Count" Skill for at least 20 minutes each day (see page 87).

2. **"One Fun a Day!"** Use one of your Fun Menus to do at least one enjoyable activity each day (if that is too much, do at least two to three in a week). XTRA FUN CREDIT - Do some **"Laughing"** every day. Find something to make you laugh for at least 30-minutes (see page 159).

3. **"Resting in Bed."** Continue using this Moving Skill to improve your night-time rest and sleep (see page 92).

4. **Catch Triggers**. Continue to identify Triggers as they come along and use Comfort Skills to disarm them and reduce pain flares and emotional upset. (see page 81).

Solving Pain Problem #5 –
"Negative Thoughts"

The Problem: You're plagued by negative thoughts that relentlessly drive you into emotional distress and harmful habits – both of which increase pain. This is because your situation often brings on these thoughts and you unknowingly follow them down the road to miserable places.

Solve it with the Re-Thinking Strategy

"Re-Thinking Strategy" is the practice of moving your thinking process away from forgetfulness and negativity and towards positive well-being. It includes two forms: 1) Re-Thinking Memory, and 2) Re-Thinking Negative Thoughts. In this Brief Training, you'll learn about the second form.

As a wise man once said, "Whatever is on your mind, that's where you are." [39] The way you think has a profound effect on your mind and body. Problems of pain, illness, depression, and other difficulties get better or worse, depending on how you think about them. For example, if you take a hopeless view of pain, you might believe that your situation is an unending story of suffering, helplessness, and loss. Such beliefs and thoughts will increase your Misery level and often cause negative events to happen (i.e., a bout of depression or panic).

By "Re-Thinking" and moving away from Negative Thoughts, you can make life better despite your painful challenges. By focusing on neutral or positive things in your life, you empower yourself to take control of your mind and brain. From there, you'll find opportunities to reduce your Misery and change some of the problems you face.

Learn/About Negative Thoughts

A **"Negative Thought"** *is any idea, belief, point of view, judgment, or mental image that increases your misery when you make it your focus of attention.* When you're dealing with Chronic Pain, you're likely to experience emotional discomfort. As I suggested in Chapter Two, you can imagine that this is brought on by "Bad Guys," such as Anxiety, Rage, and Depression, who send Negative Thoughts into your head. These create and worsen uncomfortable moods and body sensations. For example, Depression often likes to attack you with the harmful thought "I have no life." Unfortunately, if you believe this, you'll end up feeling quite low. Here is a Story Box that illustrates how Negative Thoughts may function in your life. [40]

---

[39] Rabbi Israel Ba'al Shem Tov, 18th Century.
[40] Story by Rabbi Nachman of Bratislav, see "Chassidic Masters and their Teachings," by Aryeh Kaplan.

STORY BOX #4 - Following Nothing

As a woman walked through town one day, she came across a stranger who held up a closed hand and said,

"In my hand is something that will change your life for the better. Do you want to see it?"

She said "yes" and followed him down the street, where he eventually came across a young man. The stranger held his fist up again and said,

"I have a wondrous thing in my hand that will positively change this woman's life and it can also change yours - would you like to see it?"

The young fellow agreed, and now the stranger had two people following him up one street and down another. After a while, he picked up ten more people with his promise. Eventually, he stopped walking and facing his little group he said,

"Okay, here is what you were all waiting to see."

He opened his hand and they saw...nothing. His hand was empty. The guy laughed and ran off. These people eventually realized that this trickster got them to follow him up one street and down another for nothing.

Following Negative Thoughts

Just like the trickster in the story above, destructive thoughts have no power over you unless you follow them. These toxic ideas work like con men on the street who try to manipulate you into seeing things their way. When you follow them, they lead to emotional places you don't want to go.

What can you do to prevent Negative Thoughts from making you miserable? You can "Re-Think" your situation. The Re-Thinking Skill described below will help you to *"catch harmful thoughts before they catch you."* Versions of this and other Re-thinking Skills were starting to develop over half a century ago by professional psychotherapists and researchers.[41] You can use the Skill to prevent yourself from following Negative Thoughts.

---

[41] See "Handbook of Cognitive-Behavioral Therapies – Third Edition" by Keith S Dobson (Editor).

Catastrophizing – Particularly Nasty Negative Thinking

This is a very common way that we engage in negative thinking. **"Catastrophizing"** *is a style of thinking which convinces you that events and situations are much worse than they really are.* Catastrophizing thoughts anxiously shout at us on the inside trying to convince us that something bad is going to happen and that it will be an all-out disaster! Too often, they are wrong – true, we may experience an uncomfortable situation, but it may not be a bad as we think. For example, I once worked with a person in knee pain who feared walking. Whenever I suggested it, she said, "Oh no! Last time I did that, I was in bed for a week!" I suggested that she only take ten steps away from and back towards her front door. When she came back the next week, she told me that at first she noticed lots of catastrophic thoughts telling her she would fall down or become severely flared. However, she kept walking and, after she returned home, she noticed that her knees only ached for a few minutes. In fact, the next day, they felt better.

Aside from scaring us away from healthy activities, catastrophizing thoughts often increase our Misery level and physical hurt. Like the Misery brought on by depressing or anxious thoughts, catastrophizing ideas can eventually stress you so much that your nervous system becomes more sensitive to pain. This is why it is most important to avoid this kind of thinking. As you do, Comfort can get stronger.

One way to prevent these thoughts from harassing you is to be on the lookout for them. The skill in this training will help you distance yourself from catastrophizing. To review, these thoughts have two parts and, as you become aware of them, you can better reduce them:

Part 1 – Catastrophizing thoughts tell you that something bad will happen (i.e., they, "if you take a little walk, you'll get a big pain flare")

Part 2 – They also exaggerate the "bad thing" into an utter disaster (i.e., they say, "you won't survive the flare and you'll be in bed for four months!)

Do It Now!

Re-Thinking Skill – "See it Coming"

As I've discussed earlier, Bad Guys like Depression and Pain influence you by sending negative messages into your head. If you follow these thoughts, they'll lead you into experiences that you probably want to avoid (i.e., depressed mood, increased pain awareness, over-eating, muscle tension). Cognitive-Behavioral psychologists and other practitioners have created a variety of Skills that help you notice and interrupt Negative Thoughts and harmful attitudes.

I call one of these **"See it Coming,"** and it helps you to catch destructive thoughts before they have a chance to seduce you into following them. As you notice their irritating patterns and harmful messages, you'll stop them in their tracks and prevent a lot of Misery.

STORY BOX #5 - The Snowball Demon

Jacob, a friend of mine, told me that he first learned how to "See it Coming" from his ten-year-old cousin Arnie, the "snowball demon." He'd visit Arnie in wintertime Colorado and, a usual, they'd get into a snowball fight, which ended with Arnie burying Jacob under an avalanche of ice. However, when Jake turned thirteen, he began to notice <u>how</u> Arnie threw his "snowball sandwiches."

Jacob noticed which direction the balls came from, where they hit, the faces Arnie would make before he threw one, how he stood, how big the balls were, etc. After a short while, and a lot of snowballs, he could predict where the balls would go and he easily avoided them. After that, Arnie ate all the snowball sandwiches!

Just as Jacob saw the snowballs coming, you can see Negative Thoughts coming and take action to block them. When Depression sends his sad and hopeless messages into your head, he wants you to believe that they come from you. That's what makes the thoughts so believable. You can separate yourself from these hurtful ideas by reminding yourself that, for the most part, you didn't have a lot of Negative Thoughts before Pain and other Bad Guys entered your life (or at least not as many. The next Re-Thinking Info Box will be followed by this Skill Box.

INFO BOX #15 -
Common Negative Thoughts

❖ "I'm such a cripple."
❖ "This will never change."
❖ "My life is over."
❖ "It's going to get me no matter what I do!"
❖ "I'm such a burden on everyone."

RE-THINKING SKILL BOX #2 -
"See it Coming"

Step One - Notice Them. Over the next week or two, each time you notice that you're in a low mood or anxious state, recall what kind of Negative Thoughts were rattling around in your mind before you felt bad. For example, Thoughts such as "I'm such a disappointment to others" or "I can't do anything anymore." (If that's too difficult to do when you're feeling distressed, wait until your mood improves, then recall what thoughts came along before you felt so bad).

Step Two - See It Coming with a Friendly Warning Phrase. After you've identified the Negative Thought, notice it whenever it shows up and repeat in your mind a phrase such as:

    ❖   "There he goes again!"
    ❖   "Not you again!"
    ❖   "Look who is back."
    ❖   "There's that _____ (i.e., depressing) thought from yesterday."
    ❖   "Haven't I seen you someplace before?"

Step Three - Set it Aside. After you notice the Negative Thought and say your Friendly Warning Phrase, mentally set the Thought aside and go about your daily business. If you have to repeat your Phrase several times before you can let the Thought go, that's fine.

The next story describes how one person in pain fended off the Negative Thoughts that her husband tried to put into her head.

STORY BOX #6 - Marcia Sees It Coming

I once counseled a woman named Marcia whose husband would say terrible things to make her feel guilty. Usually, they had a good relationship, but her husband's periodic "guilt tripping" was annoying the heck out of her. What's worse – she'd fall for it every time, and it left her feeling miserable and depressed. In a way, she was allowing his Negative Thoughts to enter her head.

"He gets very obnoxious and repeats the same lines over and over and I listen to it," she told me with much frustration. Marcia admitted that she wanted to stop these words from affecting her. I suggested that once she saw his guilt words coming, she could say a funny word or sentence quietly in her mind, then ignore him. Soon after our session, her husband came home and told her, "You never get dinner to the table on time and you know how this throws off our family schedule!" She immediately "Saw it Coming," and recognized that this was the same old stuff he'd throw at her when he was tired and cranky from his day. She then said to herself, "There he goes again!" and laughed about this a little on the inside. When Marcia continued preparing dinner and ignored his tantrum, he quieted down.

Later she told me that this Skill worked like a charm and it prevented Guilt from bringing her down. What was even better - as she continued to meet her husband's guilt tripping with this Re-Thinking Skill, he did it less and less.

Although this example involved a real person, you can do the same with the Negative Thoughts themselves by using the "See it Coming" Skill to disarm them. When you do this, you may experience two things:

- ❖ **First**, you'll feel more in control because you caught the thought before it caught you.
- ❖ **Second**, you might laugh at the thought and at the Bad Guy who sent it. As you giggle on the inside, perhaps you'll say things to yourself like "There he goes again, what an obnoxious Butt-head! Does Anxiety really think he can get away with that lie again!"

Overall, the more you "See it Coming," the easier it gets to catch a Negative Thought before it catches you.

RE-THINKING HOMEWORK BOX

1. **Breath Counting.** Practice the "Breath Count" for at least 20 minutes each day (see page 87).

2. **"See it Coming."** Use the Re-Thinking Skill Box above to identify some of the most common Negative Thoughts that go through your mind. Write these in a journal or a digital file for later reference. As you notice them, they can grow quieter.

3. **Enjoying Skills.** Continue "Doing Fun" in order to help your nervous system calm and your Comfort rise (see page 96).

4. **"Resting in Bed."** Continue using this Moving Skill as needed to improve your night-time rest and sleep (see page 92).

Solving Pain Problem #6 – "Distressed by Annoying People"

The Problem: There are people in your life that you relate with regularly, some of whom you deeply know and love. Unfortunately, at times, they hurt you with their criticizing, manipulating, or intimidating words and actions. You may experience some of the same problems from people you don't know very well and, unfortunately, you may believe their hurtful words and give in to their unreasonable demands.

Solve it with the Relating Strategy

"Relating Strategy" *is the practice of both increasing your positive connections to people and setting limits on those who annoy you*. We all relate – with ourselves, with people, with the environment and, for some of us, with our Spiritual Source. One definition of the word "relating" is "connecting with someone." Skills in this Strategy empower you to revive your previous social life and create new relationships. There is a growing body of research that suggests that building a positive social life improves your physical and emotional health.[42] (You can learn more about how to increase your social life in Chapter Eight, Week 6, First Training Day.)

Relationships are a wonderful thing to develop and grow; however, they can also challenge you. On the one hand, it is important to get closer to people you know and to connect with new friends, when these relationships are mutually respectful. On the other hand, when people treat you badly, the pain is likely to rise. As that happens, you can make your way back to Comfort by setting limits on the bad behavior of these "Annoying People." Below, you'll learn about 1) the effect of hurtful words and actions on your body and mind, and 2) how you can reduce or stop them.

---

[42] See "Love and Survival: Eight Pathways to Intimacy and Health" by Dean Ornish, MD.

STORY BOX #7 –
Jerry's Daily Argument

Jerry, an ex-truck driver with a very painful low-back, was in a terrible marriage with a wife who'd constantly criticize him for every little thing he did. She'd nag him endlessly, saying things like, "You take too many pain pills, You don't do enough for the house, You don't spend enough time with me, You did this and that, You didn't do this and that, and Blah, Blah, Blah..." Despite all of his efforts, he could do nothing right in her eyes. Too often, Jerry allowed her nagging to pull him into an argument that would end up sending him into a major pain flare and bruised feelings.

Learn/About Annoying People, Toxic Talk and Saying "No!"

What is an Annoying Person?

Most of us have known people who annoy us. According to the dictionary, the word "annoy" means to "disturb, harass, and irritate." **"Annoying People"** *are individuals you know (and may love) whose behavior and words make you feel uncomfortable and upset.* They are usually people who are close to you, like spouses, kids, family, friends, or neighbors. Others may include doctors, co-workers, or supervisors. Consider two types:

1. **Annoying People**. These folks may bother you occasionally (i.e., at bedtime), or regarding particular issues (i.e., finances, pain medication). Most of the time, you get along fairly well. Some of them annoy you from a place of good intentions (i.e., one husband who wouldn't let his wife do anything around the house in order to protect her from pain). Whether they disturb you a little or a lot, the annoyance is limited.

2. **Seriously Annoying People.** These guys harass you most of the time. They often unknowingly push you into a full blown argument, rage, depression, or panic attack. They might also irritate you on purpose. Some have a long history of annoying you, while others only began to treat you badly since chronic pain came into your life. Overall, you share very few happy or comfortable moments together.

The Skills in the Workbook will help with both types. However, when it comes to Seriously Annoying People, you may have to make long-term changes in order to find some happiness. No matter the type, Annoying People may include:

- A spouse who talks down to you
- A mother or father who frequently criticizes your adult choices

- A child or teenager who never does any house chores and then hits you with an argument when you ask them to do something

Regardless of how long they've bothered you, each time they do it, your nervous system may become over-stimulated, your muscles tighten, and your mood sinks down. All of these effects lead to more stress, upset, and pain.

Reasoning with the Unreasonable

Annoying People will speak or act unreasonably towards you. When they do this, they are often acting like a little two-year-old in a large body using a wide vocabulary. This means that when you try to reason with them as a mature adult, they'll answer you like a petulant child, ignoring your good intentions and attacking you for your efforts. Or, they may talk down to you as if you were a child. If you continue to try negotiating with them, you'll make ***one of the biggest mistakes you can make with these people: Attempting to reason with them when they are unreasonable.*** When you make this mistake, you'll find yourself stuck in a harmful pattern that repeats itself again and again like a bad TV re-run – you may feel like you are hitting your head against the wall.

The Painful Relationship Pattern

It goes something like this: The Annoying Person says something hurtful, you may nicely try to talk with them about it, and they answer you with more insults, manipulations, and/or emotional outbursts. You try to respond reasonably and the cycle starts over again. For example, one woman with a terrible back condition was pressured by her boyfriend to cook dinner for him every night (without his help). She tried to reasonably talk him out of it for 30 minutes to no avail. He kept nagging her and this filled her with feelings of guilt. Here, a reasonable person (the woman) tried to have a sincere conversation with someone who is unreasonable (the boyfriend). In the end, she felt miserable and gave in to his demands. You can guess what happened – each night after dinner, she suffered a severe pain flare.

What Does an Annoying Person Want?

- ❖ **Annoying people want to get their way.** For example, they'll manipulate you to feel guilty in order to get you to do something they want. Usually, it's something that you don't feel comfortable with (i.e., hiking 5 miles), or they may burden you with too many tasks and then refuse to help (i.e., expect you to clean the entire house).
- ❖ **Annoying people crave your attention.** This is big. It's highly valued by young people and adults alike. You may have observed that the more attention you give them while they are annoying you, the nastier they'll get and the longer they will bother you.

❖ **Annoying people want to invalidate you by arguing that they are right and you are wrong**. Like most people, you hold valid beliefs and take actions that are meaningful to you. Annoying people love to invalidate your beliefs and actions by demanding that their way of seeing things is right and yours is not.

When they achieve any or all of these goals, you'll most likely feel angry, upset, and hurt.

Like the Person, Hate the Behavior

Let me make something very clear – <u>Annoying People are still people</u>. The above descriptions are intended to denigrate the people who make themselves annoying. Annoying People may irritate you all (or even most) of the time, nor are they all fully aware about what they are doing. Many of them are fine people with whom you usually have good interactions. However, sometimes they have a tendency to talk to you in a hurtful manner. In the end, it is very important that you like the person (if possible) and hate their bad behavior. (This doesn't necessarily apply to "Seriously Annoying People.")

Avoid Harmful Habit #3 – "Taking in Toxic-Talk" [43]

"Toxic Talk" *is the kind of message you receive from people who criticize, manipulate, threaten, guilt trip, and generally bad mouth you. Often, these words cause you to feel very uncomfortable.* When you "give in" and allow yourself to listen to their negative words you'll end up feeling upset. What's worse, as I've suggested in this training, when you feel emotionally distressed your nervous system becomes more sensitive to pain. <u>When you spend too much time listening to the Annoying Person's poisonous words, you unintentionally allow them to put their Negative Thoughts into your head – and that hurts your body!</u>

Toxic-Talk is Poisonous

That's right. It can hurt you even more than the pain because it poisons your body. How does that happen? It's no secret that Annoying People (and especially Seriously Annoying People) will stress you out. If you allow yourself to listen to their disturbing words or yelling day after day, you'll experience high levels of chronic stress, and this causes your body to fill up with lots of stress hormones turning your body into a bowl of "Stress Hormone Soup." (Your body is already overly stressed by pain and other difficulties.) When that occurs, your health becomes compromised. If your stress level stays high on a regular basis, it can cause or worsen diseases like high blood pressure or diabetes.[44] Toxic Talk also increases your pain level and also causes emotional harm, like feelings of abandonment and guilt.

---

[43] An annotated list of twelve "Harmful Habits" that many people-in-pain do are found in Appendix B.

[44] You may find the following useful sources of information on stress and stress-related diseases: Read "Why Zebras Don't Get Ulcers" by Robert Sapolsky; also see http://en.wikipedia.org/wiki/Stress-related_disorders

In order to avoid the stress, pain, and disease that come from the hurtful words of Annoying People, **you need to walk away from them!** The longer you listen, the more poison you'll take into your system. When you stop "Taking in Toxic Talk," you protect yourself from its painful consequences.

Dealing with Annoying People

Unless you feel that it's time to leave (i.e., as often happens in the case of a Seriously Annoying Person), the most important thing to do is set a limit on their bad behavior. Effective limits do not involve rage. If you scream or make hurtful accusations back at the Annoying Person, you may end up harming yourself. Save your energy and passion for better pursuits and just firmly say "No!" to what they are doing to you. It's this kind of change that will improve your relationship over the long run. The Skills described below with help you do that.

Say "No!" to Annoying People

The Relating Skill provided in this section can help you to:

- ❖ Say "No!" to the unreasonable demands of Annoying People
- ❖ Say "No!" to their manipulation and guilt tripping
- ❖ Say "No!" to their criticisms and threats

A friend of mine once told me that "No!" is the new "Yes." You'll find that when you say "No!" to Toxic Talk and the Misery it causes, you'll also say "Yes!" to increased physical and emotional Comfort. The Relating Box that shows you how to do this will come after the following story.

STORY BOX #8 –
Monique Says "No!"

Despite the searing pain that 45-year-old Monique felt in her left foot, she was still able to work part-time as a receptionist in a large medical office. She was a very good worker and took on more than just receptionist duties. This was because, in order to save money on additional staff, her office manager expected her to take on more work than she was required. She was afraid to refuse him.

Several times a week, she'd lift and carry heavy boxes and stack forms on high shelves, causing her a lot of pain. A number of times when one of her supervisor's favorite employees gave him a last-minute request for time off, he'd ask/demand Monique to come into work on her day off. Each time he did this, she'd give in with little complaint. However, later on, her stress level intensified and this resulted in a terrible pain flare. On top of that, when she tried to call in sick after one of these flares, her supervisor would give her a hard time on the phone and pressure her to come in that day. Since she was afraid she'd lose her job, Monique would go to work in a flare and squirm all day in a chair of pain.

After she told us this sad story in the Comfort Workshop, the group members gave her a great deal of support to stand up for her rights. They also told her that she was his best, and most dependable, worker, one who is very difficult to replace. This encouraged her to deal with her manager differently.

Monique didn't have to wait long to test this out because at the end of the next day, her boss told her he needed her to stay "a little longer." Amazingly...she said, "No!" At first, he was taken aback. Then, he launched into a long, rambling speech about her obligations to their department. She knew there was no reasoning with him and so she cut him off, saying, "Sorry, Ralph, I can't do that anymore. I'm going home, see you tomorrow." She turned around and walked out, leaving him with his jaw hanging down to the floor. She did the same thing on a couple of other occasions and eventually he stopped asking. After that, her job became a much more comfortable place to work.

Two Ways to Say "No!" – Direct and Indirect Limit Setting

Two Skill-Sets empower you to firmly and effectively say "No!" to Toxic Talk.

1. The **Direct Limit Skill-Set** provides you with Skills that help you meet the challenges these people put before you. It arms those of you who are prepared to directly confront and set limits on the annoying behavior. The Skill provided below is Direct Limit Setting.

2. The **Indirect Limit Skill-Set** does this in a powerfully round-about fashion. It's for those of you who find it too difficult to directly confront the offending individual. It's made up of subtle tactics that disarm the offending person in a way that is not obvious to them. (This may work pretty well even if they are aware of what you are doing.) I offer three of these Skills in the eight-week Basic Training Course described later on in Chapter Eight.

WARNING!!! – Be Cautious with Annoying People in Power

Some Annoying People have the power to harm you financially, emotionally, or physically (i.e., your boss at work, a controlling husband who manages the bank account). If you are in a vulnerable position you should seek the advice of a counselor, a therapist, a lawyer, or the police before confronting the Annoying Person. Reserve the use of the Skills described here for people who will not seriously harm you.

Do It Now!

Relating Skill – "The C.A.L.M. Nice Guy Approach"

This Skill is very effective with people who are willing to change their behavior when you ask them to stop abusing you. These folks need a little reminder about what you'll do if they don't stop their Toxic Talk. If you're prepared to firmly (and effectively) stand up to an Annoying Person and their bad words and behavior, then this is the right Skill for you.

RELATING SKILL BOX #3 -
"The C.A.L.M. Nice Guy Approach"

Step One – Ask Yourself the "Personal 1-2-3." Annoying kids and adults confront you with their "1-2-3" → 1) I want, 2) what I want, 3) when I want it. A powerful way to counter this is with your own 1-2-3. When someone is annoying you, ask yourself the following:

- *One – "What Do I Want?"* This is critical and we often forget to ask ourselves this. Example Answers – "I want him to stop criticizing me," or, "I want her to stop asking me how I feel."
- *Two – "When Do I Want it to Happen?"* What are your time needs? Right now? In an hour? When you spell this out for yourself you leave no wiggle room for the Annoying Person to change the time.
- *Three – "What Will I Do if I Don't Get It?"* You can create and impose <u>consequences</u> on the offending person if they don't comply with your request. Examples:
  - ➤ Remove your attention by walking away
  - ➤ Briefly take away a misbehaving child's privileges (i.e., I-Pad)

Step Two – Use the C.A.L.M. Nice Guy Approach. Carry out your own "Personal 1-2-3."

C*ut Off.* Interrupt the person talking. If you don't stop the Toxic Talk, it will go on and on. Although this may feel like an impolite interruption, it's not. Useful Cut-Off lines include:

- "Excuse me."
- "Let's stop for a moment."
- "Wait! I have to tell you something."

You can even hold your hand up as if you are stopping traffic.

A*lert & Ask.* Briefly **Alert** them by saying that their words are irritating, frustrating, or hurtful. Then, **Ask** them in a sentence or two what you clearly want from them. For example:

- "You're words are upsetting me right now" (<u>Alert</u>), and
- "I want you to stop talking to me that way right now" (<u>Ask</u>)

Limit. Add to the end of your request a warning that if you don't get what you're asking for, you may have to do something they won't like – usually removing your attention from them by walking away. You can phrase the Limit using an **"If - Then Statement,"** said either in the negative or positive:

- *Negative Example* - **"If** you don't stop criticizing me, **Then** I'm going out for a while by myself."
- *Positive Example* - **"If** you stop criticizing me, **Then** we can talk."

Move On to Something Good. If the person doesn't stop their Toxic Talk or upsetting behavior, the discussion is **OVER**. No more talking or reasoning with them. Tell them that you'll see them later and then "Move On" by walking away for a while. How do you do this? – Turn around and follow your feet! But that is not all – in order to clean out any bad feelings caused by their Toxic Talk, its best to do something enjoyable. The more upset you are, the bigger the pleasure you deserve. You can return to the person later, when they've either apologized or begun to speak to you with more respect and care.

"Fly-Fishing" Alert!!

If you have to walk away, the Annoying Person may try to pull you back into the argument with lines like "There you go, leaving again!" or "What kind of wife/husband are you!?" Don't fall for this "fly fishing" – just follow your feet out of the room and "Move on to Something Good."

STORY BOX #9 –
Cindy Stays C.A.L.M.

Cindy's father was always nagging her about her work habits. Since she survived a car accident three years ago, Cindy changed her way of carrying out her tasks. She worked for a publishing company as an editor and her boss allowed her to do book editing assignments in her home and at her own pace. She'd work at her home computer station and take a lot of breaks. This allowed her to feel more Comfort over the constant pain she felt in her back.

113

Unfortunately, this wasn't good enough for her father, a "self-made-man" who advanced in his company to become a vice-president for sales. Again and again, on the phone or face-to-face, he'd bring up how she "should be more active" and "go to work like everybody else." Most times, Cindy came away from his nagging sessions exhausted and depressed. Sometimes, she yelled back at him and this made things worse.

When Cindy learned about the C.A.L.M. Skill, she decided to use it on her father to stop his Toxic Talk. One Monday, he came to her house for a visit and found her taking a break on her recliner. Seeing this, he began to criticize her for being "lazy." Cindy "Saw it Coming," continued sitting comfortably in her chair, and did the following:

- *Cut Off.* Holding up her hand, she said, "Dad, wait a minute."
- *Alert & Ask.* "When you criticize me like that, I feel very bad and it does not help me to work or feel comfortable. I'd like you to stop talking about how I work and change the subject to something more positive."
- *Limit.* "If you can do that, then I want you to stay and we can have a nice visit. But, if you feel that you have to keep criticizing me and telling me what to do, then let's stop talking now and I'll see you later."
- *Move on to Something Good.* Sadly, her father could not respect her request, so she told him to leave. Even though she felt relief from his nagging, she felt bad about the interaction they had. To return herself to a happier state, she decided to accept that she'd feel bad for a while. While she waited for the mood to pass, she took a nice walk and then watched a funny video.

Later, Cindy told me that this Skill worked like a charm and it prevented her father and Guilt from bringing her down. What was even better - as she continued to meet her dad's guilt-tripping with this Relating Skill, he annoyed her less and less.

RELATING HOMEWORK BOX

1. **Breath Counting.** Practice the "Breath Count" Skill for at least 20 minutes each day (see page 87).

2. **Relating Skill: Say "No!"** Review the "C.A.L.M. Approach" described above. Imagine applying it to a recent situation you've had with an Annoying Person. Eventually, put the Skill into practice with that person the next time they speak badly to you. (REMEMBER: Make sure that this is safe to do.)

3. **Enjoying Skill.** Use this Skill to have fun every day (see page 95).

4. **"Resting in Bed."** Use this Moving Skill to improve your night-time rest and sleep (see page 91).

Bonus: Solving Pain Problem #7 – "Underprepared for Pain Flares"

The Problem: When pain flares come, you feel unprepared to handle them and that adds to the hurt and upset. When you're caught off guard, you're likely to feel helpless and you might panic.

Solve it with the Moving Strategy – Pain Flare Planning

A **"Pain Flare"** *is an intense, and sometimes sudden, increase in your physical discomfort.* If you're unprepared for a pain flare, you're likely to feel helpless and you might panic. These reactions may cause you even more hurt and upset. Overall, you may feel unprepared to handle chronic pain and Misery, and this reinforces the false idea that you have no control over your life. On the contrary, you can take charge by planning what you'll do during a flare.

Fire Drills and Flare Plans

Remember when you were a kid in Elementary School and the fire bell rang? Your teacher would quickly line you up and firmly instruct you to exit the classroom and walk to a safe place. (Like most school children, you were probably excited to get out of class for a while!) Fire Drills are a normal part of most educational institutions and they help children to reduce their anxiety during times when they're faced with an emergency situation. Escape plans and drills are also helpful for adults by preparing them to handle a fire or natural disasters such as earthquakes and hurricanes.

A pain flare is another kind of emergency situation. All of you know that the daily pain level you live with is bad enough without pain flares. As suggested above, when pain intensifies, it can drive you into a state of panic and emotional distress. Just as you follow an escape plan in the case of fire, you can follow another plan that helps you to reduce or at least better tolerate a pain flare. It's very empowering because when the discomfort suddenly elevates, you won't need to think up any solutions on the spot – just follow your Plan. As you do this, you'll return to a better level of Comfort and diminish some of the discomfort caused by these temporary attacks.

Do It Now!

Moving Skill – "Flare Planning in Sets of Three"

Just as there are many ways to set a goal, there are many formats you can use to create your own Flare Plan. Although these run the gamut from very basic to very comprehensive, I lean more toward the simple and straightforward. The Plan format below includes a combination of the Comfort Skills as well as practices you've developed yourself. After the next story, I'll detail options to creating a Pain Flare Plan in a Skill Box.

STORY BOX #10 –
Carolyn's "Comfort Box"

Carolyn is a retired bank officer who came to see me a number of years ago. She is one of many people in this country who suffer from chronic low back pain and depression. In the past, when a flare came along, she'd writhe in a tortured bed of pain for at least two excruciating days. The increased pain intensity often pushed past the effect of her medication, which offered little relief. After some months attending my ongoing Comfort Circle support group, Carolyn carried a very large boot box in to a session. As she opened it up, she said, "This is my Comfort Box. I decided to make a Flare Plan that I could hold in my hands, so I put this together. It sits by my bed-stand and I only open it when the pain flares up. It has many of the things I enjoy - special CD's and DVD's, a Bible, chocolates, books, a list of people to send letters and emails to, a list of people to call for casual conversations, and a list of things I can look up on the Internet. As I rest up from the flare, I use these things to distract me from the pain and, most of the time, I feel more relaxed and in control."

Everyone in the group thought that the Comfort Box was a great idea and some made their own. Carolyn continues to use her Box and gets a lot of help from it.

MOVING SKILL BOX #7 –
"Flare Planning in Sets of Three"

Step One - List Your Skills. Recall what practices you've done in the past that brought you some relief. Write them down in a journal or a digital file.

Step Two - Add New Comfort Skills to the List. Next, look over the Comfort Skills found in this book and choose those that have been effective for you (see Chapter Three). Add them to your list.

Step Three - Organize the Top Nine into Sets of Three. Look over your list and choose nine of the most helpful Skills and personal resources. Follow this format:

    A) Using your journal, or a digital file, list these nine into sets of three, with the most useful sets towards the top.

    B) Choose another nine and organize them the same way. Repeat this again and again until you have a collection of several "Sets of Three."

    C) Transfer this Flare Plan to something you can carry with you (i.e., a 3x5 card, small calendar, or a smart phone).

    D) (If you're not sure what Comfort Skills to use, choose from my sample Pain Flare Plan below.)

Step Four – Rehearse the Plan. Choose a time when you're not in a pain flare and rehearse your Plan in your mind. Imagine that the pain is flaring up and mentally experience yourself using each of the Skills in Sets of Three (i.e., Imagine you are watching something funny on your I-Pad or TV).

Final Step –Use it for a Real Pain Flare. When you notice the First Sign of an impending flare, or if you've already begun to flare, pull out your list and begin to practice the Skills in the first Set of Three. After thirty minutes, if you're not comfortable enough, practice another Set of Three or repeat some on the first Set. Use as many Skills as you wish.

Remember
- Don't try to get rid of the pain, let it be there and focus on practicing the Skill. Allow the Comfort to come in its own time.

EXAMPLE BOX
"SETS OF THREE FLARE PLAN"

SITUATION – *You are washing the dishes and you feel a very intense and sharp ache in your shoulder. You recall that this usually warns you that a flare is on the way* (a First Sign). *Since you know that a full blown pain flare might be coming, you decide to take out your Flare Plan and practice the "Sets of Three" until you feel more at ease.*

The Flare Plan

Set Number One
1) *"Pay as You Go"* – Take a break from the dishes and rest
2) *"Breath Count"* – Sit in a comfortable seat and practice for 15 minutes
3) *"Laughing"* – Watch a comedy DVD for at least 30 minutes

Set Number Two
1) *"Doing Fun"* – Take a hot bath
2) After the bath, do some gentle stretches for 15 minutes
3) *"The Head Trip"* – Practice for at least 15 minutes (perhaps imagining that you are on a beautiful Island sunning yourself on the beach)

Set Number Three
1) Call someone you'd love to talk with
2) *Positive Distraction – "The Fast Menu"* – Surf the Internet for 30 minutes, or walk, bike or drive to a pretty place, park somewhere, and "people-watch"
3) *"Mantra/Breath Meditation"* – For 20 minutes, practice pairing a word (i.e., "calm") to your breath. Sound it out quietly in your mind with each exhale

Remember
▪ **Keep your Flare Plan handy;** put it where you can get to it. After a while, you may have memorized parts of it and you won't need to look at it as often.

▪ **Replace *desperate searching* for pain relief with *calm curiosity*.** Notice what happens after you use a Skill and allow the Comfort to come in its own time.

HOMEWORK AND SKILL REVIEW BOX
FOR THE REST OF YOUR LIFE

1. **Breath Counting.** Use Re-Focusing Box #1 to practice the "Breath Count" Skill for at least 20 minutes daily (see page 87).

2. **Make a Flare Plan.** Create your own "Sets of Three" Flare Plan. Use it to help you ride out high levels of pain. XTRA CREDIT – Put together your own Comfort Box of enjoyable distractions.

3. **Noticing Negatives.** Identify Triggers that set off pain and emotional upsets. When you notice any, draw on other Comfort Skills to help you disarm them (see page 81).

4. **"Rest in Bed."** Use other Comfort Skills to improve your night-time rest and sleep (see page 92).

5. **"One Fun a Day!"** Do at least one thing each day that you enjoy. Build a Fun Menu (see page 95).

6. **"See it Coming."** Identify some of the most common Negative Thoughts that go through your mind. Write these in your Journal or digital file for later reference (see page 102).

7. **Say "No!"** Review the Relating Skill on page 112 and imagine applying it to a difficult interaction you've had with an Annoying Person. Eventually, use the Skill when that person speaks badly to you. (REMEMBER – make sure that you are safe before using that Skill.)

Chapter Eight – The Eight-Week Basic Training Course

Table of Contents

Week Seven – Dealing with Annoying People & Hypnosis

Week Eight – Comfort Skill Review & Seeing a New Future

Basic Training Introduction

The best option you have to develop a more comfortable life is YOU. The actions you take will make the difference. In this training course, you will have the opportunity to learn thirty-six Comfort Skills that empower you to resolve thirteen Pain Problems commonly experienced by people-in-pain. As you use these Skills, you'll increase your Comfort level, which will either reduce the pain or help you to "ride it out" with more ease.

The course presents the Comfort Skills in eight weekly training sections. If you decide that all eight weeks are too much to take on now, you can either move slowly through the course or use shorter "Brief Training" in Chapter Seven. Please feel free to engage in this training any way you wish.

Pain Problems –The Miserable Thirteen

As I discussed in Chapter Four, chronic pain is often accompanied by a number of challenges. These **"Pain Problems"** *are pain-related difficulties that increase your Misery and pain levels.* They include common troubles such as poor sleep and low moods and often co-occur with chronic pain. Research over the last few decades shows that when these Problems are left unsolved, they can add to your Misery and raise your discomfort (i.e., a poor night's sleep makes you feel miserable and achy in the morning). The next Info Box briefly reviews thirteen of these Misery-causing Problems that are addressed in the Basic Training.

INFO BOX #8 –
"Thirteen Pain Problems
that Accompany Chronic Pain"

1. Unpredictable Pain Flares and Emotional Distress

2. Attention Hijacked by Pain and Stress

3. Poor Sleep and Rest at Night

4. Sadness, Worry and Other Miserable Feelings

5. Negative Thoughts

6. Distress Caused by Annoying People

7. Underprepared for Pain Flares

8. Missing the Good Things in Your Life

9. Hypersensitive Nervous System

10. No Positive Future in Sight

11. Unbalanced Activity

12. Poor Memory

13. Isolation and Loneliness

The eight weekly sections of this long chapter will show you how to solve these Problems and raise your Comfort level in a variety of ways

How is the Eight-Week Basic Training Program Organized?

At the beginning of each weekly section, you'll see a short list of the Problems and Skills included in that training. After that is a "Contents Box" for each of the three "Training Days" (see pages 121 and 122 for the complete list of Training weeks and Days). Here is how each Basic Training Day is organized:

INFO BOX – #16
TRAINING DAY FORMAT

The Skill Review. In order to develop your ability to get more Comfort, you'll most Training Days practicing one or two of the Comfort Skills you learned in previous Training Days.

Today's Pain Problems. Pain Problems addressed on a particular Training Day will be listed.

Learn/About. It's not always necessary to fully understand the reasons behind a Skill in order to benefit from its use. However, if you'd like to learn the background of some Pain Problems and Comfort Skills, this segment presents a brief description about them.

Skill of the Day. This segment provides the descriptions and instructions you'll need to practice that day's new Comfort Skills.

The Last Practice. Often, I'll introduce a new Re-Focusing Skill in this segment. I'll also invite you to practice a Skill you have learned already. As the old saying goes, "Repetition is the mother of learning."

Homework Box. In order to benefit the most from the Skills, it's best to do them regularly between Training Days. The Homework Box provides a number of suggested assignments you can practice.

Two Ways to Use the Basic Training

1) **Skill-Centered Training.** You can choose to focus your efforts on learning the Skills. Although you may not need all of them, some Skills will improve your life as you practice them. Two possible Skill-Centered routes you can take include:

   A) *Straight-Through.* Some of you like to learn a lot as soon as possible. If that learning style fits you, then follow this three-day-a-week learning sequence as it is. You might, for example, finish one Training Day on Monday, one on Wednesday, and the last on Friday.

   B) *Slow-and-Steady.* You might choose to do the training more slowly. For example, you may decide to take an entire week to learn the information and Skills in one Training Day.

2) **Problem-Centered Training.** You can consult the list of Pain Problems in Chapter Four and choose the Problems that you are interested in solving. Each one has a list of Comfort Skills below i.

The Journal

A number of Skill Boxes will instruct you to do some writing. You may find it very useful to buy a blank journal and turn it into your "Basic Training" or "Comfort Skill" Journal. You can keep a number of notes and other writings in that one book and review them from time to time.

Week One – Breathing & Goal Setting
Eight-Week Basic Training

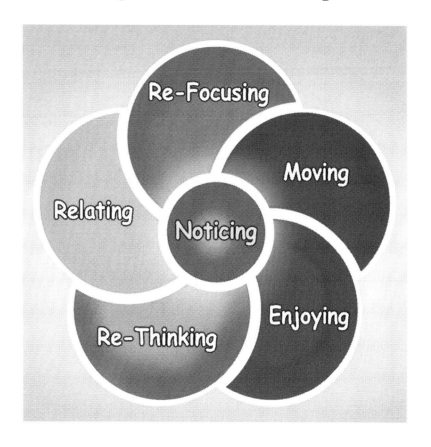

Pain Problems and Comfort Skill Solutions
Included in Week One

Pain Problems
- *"Attention Hijacked by Pain and Stress"*
- *"Hypersensitive Nervous System"*
- *"Sadness, Worry, & Other Miserable Feelings"*
- *"No Positive Future in Sight"*

Comfort Skill Solutions
- *"The Breath Count"*
- *"Set a Goal, Create a Future"*

WEEK ONE CONTENTS BOX

The Breath Count
First Training Day

1. Today's Pain Problems
   - *Pain Problem #2 – "Attention Hijacked by Pain and Stress"*
   - *Pain Problem #9 – "Hypersensitive Nervous System"*
   - *Pain Problem #4 – "Sadness, Worry, & Other Miserable Feelings"*
2. The First Skill
   A) *"Breath Count"*
3. Learn/About #1 - Pain and Comfort
4. The Last Practice
   A) *"Breath Count"*
5. Homework Box

The Breath Count and Goal Setting I
Second Training Day

1. The Skill Review
   A) *"Breath Count"*
2. Today's Pain Problem
   - *Pain Problem #10 - "No Positive Future in Sight"*
3. Learn/About #2 - The Moving Strategy
4. Learn/About #3 – The Activity Arc
5. Skill of the Day
   A) *"Set a Goal, Create a Future"* (Steps One and Two)
6. The Last Practice
   A) *"Breath Count"*
7. Homework Box

The Re-Focusing Strategy and Goal Setting II
Third Training Day

1. The Skill Review
   A) *"Breath Count"*
2. Learn/About #4 - The Re-Focusing Strategy
3. Today's Pain Problem
   - *Pain Problem #10 - "No Positive Future in Sight"*
4. Skill of the Day
   A) *"Set a Goal, Create a Future" (Step Three)*
5. The Last Practice
   A) *"Breath Count"*
6. Homework Box

The Breath Count
First Training Day – Week 1

Today's Pain Problems
Pain Problem #2 – "Attention Hijacked by Pain and Stress"
Pain Problem #9 – "Hypersensitive Nervous System"

The First Skill
"Breath Count"

We breathe all of the time. ("How good is that!?) The **"Breath Count"** Skill is a relatively easy one to use because breathing is a natural function of your body – the wonderful and convenient thing about your breath is that you carry it with you wherever you go, making it easy to use as you change your physiology and generate relief and calm. When you practice the "Breath Count," you may feel like you're counting sheep without the sheep. It comes from the Zen Meditation tradition and combines two forms of concentration: **1) Physical Concentration** (Re-Focusing on the feeling of your breath moving in and out of your belly or chest), and **2) Mental Concentration** (counting numbers silently in your mind). Scientists have demonstrated that the "Breath Count" and other forms of Meditation powerfully help you redirect your attention away from pain and towards more calm and Comfort.[45]

---

[45] "Full Catastrophe Living: Using the wisdom of the Body and the Mind to Face Stress, Pain, and Illness" by Jon Kabat-Zinn, Ph.D.

RE-FOCUSING SKILL BOX #1 –
"The Breath Count"

Step One - Quiet Place and Timer. First, find a quiet place to sit and set a timer for five (or more) minutes. Choose a seat or recliner that supports your body. Remember, if you lie down, you may fall asleep.

Step Two - Breaths in the Belly. Start with a couple of deep breaths and focus on the feeling of your belly moving in and out. Then, continue following your natural breath. If the belly is an uncomfortable place to focus on, choose another part of your body (i.e., hands), and imagine the breath moving in and out of there.

Step Three - Breath Count. As you breathe naturally, count each exhale quietly in your mind. After ten breaths, start again at one. If you lose count, simply start with the number one. <u>Variation</u> – as you inhale, think the word "and" (i.e., inhale - "and," exhale - "one"). Continue counting each cycle of ten until your practice time is up.

Step Four - Returning. After the timer goes off, take three slow, deep breaths and as you exhale for the third time, allow your eyes to slowly open. Take time to "awaken" from the experience; walk around a little.

Remember - Let Distractions Be There and Re-Focus

When a distracting thought, memory, image, feeling, sound, or anything tries to move your mind away from the breath, <u>let it be there and return your mind back to focus</u>. Don't fight the distractions; simply re-focus your attention back to the breath and the count.

Learn/About #1 – Pain and Comfort

If you would like to review how pain and comfort work, please turn to Chapter One.

The Last Practice

"Breath Count"

You will discover that after you finish practicing a Re-Focusing Skill (i.e., "Breath Count"), your brain will be in a calmer state (even if you don't notice this at first). When you do the Skill again, even after an hour or so, you'll often experience that second round as a deeper, more pleasant experience than the first. Please use the Skill instructions above and practice the "Breath Count" for 5 to 10 minutes right now.

HOMEWORK BOX
FIRST TRAINING DAY – WEEK 1

The Breath Count. During the interim days before the next Training Day, practice the Breath Count at least once a day, even for 5-minutes. You might also benefit from doing a little just before you go to sleep at night (see page 130).

The Breath Count and Goal Setting I
Second Training Day – Week 1

The Skill Review

"Breath Count"

After practicing this Skill for several days, you may notice that some changes have happened. Maybe you've observed that it's just a little bit easier to focus your attention. If this isn't the case, don't worry about it; changes come in time. Until then, rustle up all of your patience and take at least 5 minutes now to repeat the "Breath Count" exercise found on page 131. Remember, avoid "trying" to make something happen. For now, "just do it to do it" and allow the Comfort, relaxation, and calm come in their own time.

Today's Pain Problem
Pain Problem #10 – "No Positive Future in Sight"

Learn/About #2 – The Moving Strategy
The **"Moving Strategy"** *is the practice of moving comfortably and confidently through four tasks which are common to people-in-pain: Goal Setting, Moving the Body, Sleep and Rest, and Pain Flare Planning.* This Training Day will introduce you to the first.

Learn/About #3 – Under-Doing

Unfortunately, some people-in-pain respond to chronic pain by engaging in "Under-Doing" - the intentional avoidance of healthy actions like walking, socializing, and carrying out the activities of daily living. It's understandable why someone in pain would avoid activities – they feel uncomfortable or miserable. Like Over-Doing, Under-Doing has several downsides, including:

    1) Increased stiffness and inflexibility in your body

    2) Physical deconditioning (being out of shape)

    3) Increased Misery and pain

The next Comfort Skill, "Set a Goal, Create a Future," shows you how to increase your activity life.

Skill of the Day

"Set a Goal, Create a Future"

A **"Goal"** *is an activity or an experience that moves you towards a new, desirable future*. Example goals can include exercise, socializing, pursuing a hobby, returning to a form of work, or practicing Comfort Skills. Here are some guidelines for choosing and pursuing a Goal:

- **Doable**. It's something that you can actually do. Be sure to avoid impossible projects (i.e., hiking up and down a mountain for three hours)
- **Relatively Comfortable**. The activity should only cause mild to moderate discomfort, which will eventually pass. For example, you might feel a bit awkward when you first meet new people – this will fade as you spend more time with them.
- **Specific**. Exactly what kind of activity do you want to do? How much time do you want to put into it? What do you want to accomplish? The more specific the goal, the easier it is to plan.
- **Approach it Slowly**. Choose a Goal you can move towards using Baby Steps (i.e., increasing your walk by five steps every other day). However, if you are comfortable moving more quickly, you can take larger steps

This next Skill Box will provide details on how to set and pursue a Goal and build a new future.

MOVING SKILL BOX #1 -
"Set a Goal, Create a Future"

Step One - Brain-Storm Goals. First, think about some possible Goals you'd like to pursue. Write them all down, even the ones that sound ridiculous. You might choose new Goals or increase your efforts to reach other goals that you're already pursuing. You may also choose something you haven't done for a while and "do it differently." Here is a short list of Goals that some of my clients have chosen:

- Exercise
- Socializing with family or friends
- Reading, study, or class attendance
- Working or volunteering
- Religious or spiritual practice

Step Two – Make a "Goal List" from Your "Brain-Storm List." Select out the most realistic goal ideas on your Brain-Storm list and build a new Goal list from them. Put them in order of interest (i.e., walking, socializing).

Step Three – Choose Your First Goal. Pick one goal from your Goal List and detail what it would look like to do. Example - if you choose a physical activity like gardening, perhaps youd decide to set aside two times a week to work on your garden for two twenty-minute sessions each day.

Step Four - Create and Record "Baby Steps." Develop some small steps you'd take towards reaching your goal (see the Example Box on next page).

Remember

➤ **"Do It Differently."** You can make your Goal doable by changing your approach to it. Example - if you used to cook an entire meal on your own before you were afflicted by pain, you may decide to invite over a person or two to help you.

➤ **Adjust It When Necessary.** Make it okay to adjust or change your Goal when necessary.

➤ **Keep Track of Your Progress.** Record your progress in a journal or digital file. Example – For a walking Goal, you might write something like this:
  - Monday, walked 15-minutes
  - Wednesday, walked 15-and-a-half-minutes

EXAMPLE BOX -
Sample Goal → "Getting More Social"

Step One - Brain-Storm Goals.

- Walking seven blocks a day
- Making new friends
- Reading more novels
- Prepare to go on a trip

Step Two – Choose One or More Goals and Make It Specific. I decided to combine a couple of Goals and came up with this one – "I want to make new friends and read more novels." To reach my Goal, I'll join a Book Club. Specifically, every two weeks, I'll meet with people in the Book Club to talk about the novel we read.

Step Three - Create & Record the Baby Steps Towards the Goal. Examples are

- Go online and look up Book Clubs in my area. Read about them for about 15 minutes.
- Do this again at another time.
- On another day, I'll write down three that look interesting.
- I'll sit, close my eyes, and think about what novels I'd like to read.
- I'll think about when and where I'll read my novel.
- I'll consider how to prepare myself for a Club meeting.
- Eventually, I'll call up one of the clubs and talk to someone about it.
- Later on I'll read one novel and go to one club meeting.

SUGGESTION BOX
Sample Goals to Pursue

1. Walking
2. Developing a new hobby
3. Exploring a new kind of paid work
4. Volunteering to work with children
5. Taking on a new Comfort Skill
6. Starting a support group
7. Learning how to paint or draw pictures
8. Writing a book, story or article
9. Studying how to play an instrument
10. Joining a chorus
11. Attend college a class
12. Become part of a religious or spiritual group
13. Participate in a monthly book club
14. Joining a Church or other religious/spiritual community
15. Attend a gentle Yoga class
16. Go on a trip
17. Read a different kind of book
18. Start an Internet business

After you finish the Last Practice below, go to the Homework Box and start working on the *"Set a Goal, Create a Future"* Skill.

The Last Practice
"Breath Count"

Practice the "Breath Count." See if you can increase your practice 10 to 15 minutes (see page 130).

HOMEWORK BOX
SECOND TRAINING DAY – WEEK 1

1. **The Breath Count.** Before the next Training Day, practice the Breath Count at least once each day. You might also benefit from doing a little just before you go to sleep (see page 130).

2. **Setting a Goal.** Do Step One and Two in the Skill Box above to develop one or more Goals that you'd like to reach by the end of a period of time (i.e., 3-months).

The Re-Focusing Strategy and Goal-Setting II
Third Training Day – Week 1

The Skill Review

"Breath Count"

Repeat the "Breath Count" and see if you can add more minutes to your practice. Remember, avoid trying to make something happen – "just do it to do it" and allow the Comfort, relaxation, and calm to come in their own time (see page 130).

Today's Pain Problem
Pain Problem #10 – "No Positive Future in Sight"

Learn/About #4 – The Re-Focusing Strategy

"Re-Focusing Strategy" *is a set of Skills that direct your attention towards something neutral or pleasant* "The Breath Count" is one of eight different Re-Focusing Skills included in this Strategy. As you develop control over your attention, you'll more easily direct it to comfortable things.

Skill of the Day

"Set a Goal, Create a Future" –
Step Three

You can continue this Skill by taking the goal you created on the previous Training Day and divide your goal-seeking tasks into "Baby Steps" (see Step Three in the Skills Box located on page 134).

The Last Practice
"Breath Count"

Practice the "Breath Count" Skill for at least fifteen minutes.

HOMEWORK BOX
THIRD TRAINING DAY – WEEK 1

1. **The Breath Count.** During the interim days before the next training week, practice the Breath Count at least once each day or night. You might also benefit from doing a little just before you go to sleep (see page 130).

2. **Continue Planning and Pursuing Your Goals**. Follow the Baby Steps you've created that lead you towards your Goals (or finish setting those Steps).

Week Two – Noticing, Laughing & the Body Bank
Eight Week Basic Training

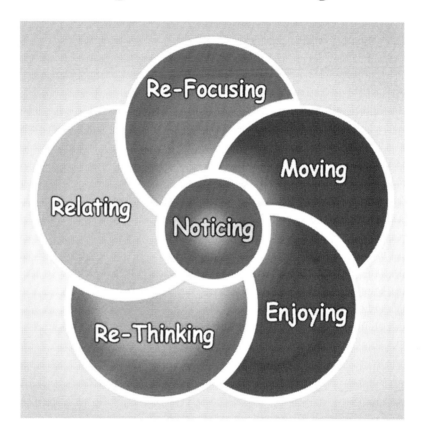

Pain Problems and Comfort Skill Solutions
Included in Week Two

Pain Problems

- *"Attention Hijacked by Pain and Stress"*
- *"Sadness, Worry, & Other Miserable Feelings"*
- *"Unpredictable Pain Flares and Emotional Distress"*
- *"Missing the Good Things in Your Life"*
- *"Unbalanced Activity Increases Pain and Stress"*

Comfort Skill Solutions

- *"Revealing Triggers"* and *"Revealing Signs"*
- *"Breath Massage"*
- *"Laughing"*
- *"Doing Fun"*
- *"I Want to See More of..."*
- *"Pay as You Go"* and *"The Payment Plan."*

WEEK TWO CONTENTS BOX

The Noticing Strategy, Negative Triggers, and First Signs
First Training Day

1. The Skill Review
   A) *"Breath Count"*
2. Today's Pain Problem
   - *Pain Problem #1 - "Unpredictable Pain Flares and Emotional Distress"*
3. Learn/About #5 - The Noticing Strategy
4. Skill of the Day
   A) *"Revealing Triggers"*
   B) *"Revealing First Signs"*
5. The Last Practice
   A) *"Breath Massage"*
6. Homework Box

Noticing Positives and Laughing Your Head Off
Second Training Day

1. The Skill Review
   A) *"Breath Massage"*
2. Today's Pain Problems
   - *Pain Problem #2 - "Attention Hijacked by Pain and Stress"*
   - *Pain Problem #4 - "Sadness, Worry, and Other Miserable Feelings"*
   - *Pain Problem #8 - "Missing the Good Things in Your Life"*
3. Learn/About #6 – The Enjoying Strategy and Enjoying Right Now
4. Learn/About #7– The Health Effects of Laughter
5. Skills of the Day
   A) *"Laughing"*
   B) *"Doing Fun"*
   C) *"I Want to See More of…"*
6. The Last Practice
   A) *"Breath Massage"*
7. Homework Box

The Comfort Account in Your "Body Bank"
Third Training Day

1. The Skill Review
   - A) *"I Want To See More of..."*
   - B) *"Breath Massage"*
2. Today's Pain Problem
   - ▪ *Pain Problem #11 - "Unbalanced Activity Increases Pain and Stress"*
3. Learn/About #8 – The Comfort Account in Your "Body Bank"
4. Skill of the Day
   - A) *"Pay as You Go – Three Options"*
   - B) *"The Payment Plan."*
5. The Last Practice
   - A) *"Breath Massage"*
6. Homework Box

The Noticing Strategy – Negative Triggers & First Signs
First Training Day – Week 2

The Skill Review

"Breath Count"
Practice the "Breath Count" Skill for at least fifteen to twenty minutes (see page 130).

Today's Pain Problem
Pain Problem #1 –
"Unpredictable Pain Flares & Emotional Distress"

Learn/About #5 – The Noticing Strategy
The first of the six Strategies on the Comfort Wheel is the **"Noticing Strategy,"** *which is the practice of making yourself aware of the positive and negative events that occur in your daily life.* The Skills in this section will show you how to notice "Negatives" that warn

142

you about a coming pain flare or stressful situation. The Noticing Strategy also includes Skills that train you to observe Positives that occur in your daily life (i.e., a fun activity, conversation with a friend). When you notice a Negative, you can use other skills to reduce its presence in your life. As you observe the Positives, they can lift your spirit and increase positive mood.

Skills of the Day Introduction

A "**Negative**" *is an event that either sets off or warns you that a pain flare or emotional upset is on the way.* Two types are "Triggers" and "First Signs."

1. "**Triggers**" *are events or situations that set off a bad mood or a pain flare* (i.e., bright lights often set off migraine headaches, or criticism can enrage you). Triggers often originate outside of you in the physical or social world. Sometimes activities can trigger you.

2. "**First Signs**" *take place inside your body and mind and warn you that a pain flare or emotional upset is coming* Its often a response to a Trigger and might include muscle tension, hopeless thoughts, depressed feeling, or over-eating.

Chicken or the Egg? – An Example

Some of you might find it difficult to tell the difference between a "Trigger" and a "First Sign." It may not always be necessary to do this. Here is one example to illustrate the differences: Let's say that you have a low-back injury, and you bend over one time to pick up something – that is an Activity Trigger. Fairly soon, you notice that your back muscles begin to tense up – that sensation is a First Sign. If you don't avoid the Trigger (bending and lifting) or you don't listen to the warning of that First Sign (muscle ache), you might bend over and lift something several times and eventually suffer from a major pain flare. In the end, it doesn't matter whether or not you define and act on something happening as a Trigger or a First Sign – as long as you notice the Negatives that come before a pain flare or upsetting emotion, you'll be able to 1) predict when a problem is coming, and 2) do something to change it. The next Info Box describes these Negatives.

INFO BOX #11 –
Negative Triggers and First Signs

Triggers. These tend to cause physical or emotional distress, which increases pain. Three broad categories include the following:

- *Physical Triggers.* Things you see or feel in your physical surroundings that cause problems. Examples – bad weather, loud noises.
- *Social Triggers.* People in your life who irritate you and worsen pain and stress. Examples – A nagging spouse or annoying co-worker.
- *Activity Triggers.* There are things you do that can set off episodes of discomfort. Examples – Lifting heavy weight or lying around a lot.

First Signs. These happen to your body and mind when you're exposed to a Trigger. First Signs warn you that a pain flare or distressing event is coming. There are five different types:

- *Physical First Signs*. Many come in the form of body sensations such as tight neck/shoulders, a rapid heartbeat, sudden fatigue, or achy feet.
- *Thought First Signs*. In reaction to a Trigger, your mind often turns to negative thoughts (i.e., When asking for help, you might think: "I'm a burden on everyone").
- *Imagined First Signs*. What you see, hear, and feel in your imagination can alert you that pain and distress are coming (i.e., imagining an argument you once had with someone).
- *Emotional First Signs*. Feelings such as anxiety, anger, and sadness warn you that you've become vulnerable to a flare.
- *Behavioral First Signs*. Some of your actions may indicate that a problem is imminent (i.e., rushing around nervously, yelling at people).

STORY BOX #2 –
The Negatives of Chocolate Cake

Thirty-five-year-old Jane suffered from damaged knees. After learning that each pound of her body weight put four pounds of pressure on her knees, she decided to go on diet. She thought that if she could lose some weight, she'd get some relief. For five months, she'd been trying to meet her goals but found that this was very difficult. One challenging moment came along one day when she felt a gnawing hunger in the pit of her stomach. The problem was that this happened right after she finished lunch! In addition to this, she also experienced thoughts that said things like, "Oh boy, a hot fudge sundae would be a great end to lunch," and "That Danish I had on Saturday was really delicious." She was also a little upset because in the morning she had a big argument with her mother on the phone. This caused her to replay angry thoughts in her head again and again, such as, "My mother is so unfair." She decided to do some housework to forget the call and she ended up doing too much, causing a moderate pain flare in her knees.

As if this wasn't bad enough, when she hobbled into the living room, she found a chocolate cake in an open bakery box sitting on the coffee table. Apparently, her husband brought a treat home for the kids. Jane looked at it for a long time and, as she tried to walk away, a sudden image flashed in her mind. She saw herself seated at the kitchen table with a glass of milk and a large chunk of chocolate cake. That was it! – she turned around and turned her fantasy into a reality by eating the cake. Suffice it to say that she didn't lose weight that day.

The next Box uses Jane's story to help you identify the Triggers and First Signs that caused her difficulties.

INFO BOX #12 –
The Negatives in Jane's Story

Jane's Triggers. These pushed her to eat fattening foods.

- *Physical Trigger.* The chocolate cake sitting on the living room table.
- *Social Trigger.* The criticizing tone and words from her mother that she heard on the phone (which stressed her out).
- *Activity Trigger.* She did too much housework and that created pain. This added discomfort made her vulnerable to use something familiar to soothe herself (i.e., the cake).

Jane's First Signs. All of the signs described below warned Jane that the urge to eat sweets was on its way.

1. *Physical First Signs*. She felt muscle tension in her shoulders after arguing with her mother. This caused her to seek relief from physical stress (i.e., by doing comfort-eating)
2. *Thought First Signs.* Jane angrily thought "My mother is so unfair!" and "A hot fudge sundae would taste good now." The first thought motivated her to seek something to calm herself and the second gave her the bad idea of what that could be.
3. *Imagined First Signs*. She imagined herself feeling better while eating chocolate cake. This is a very "dangerous" image for a person trying to diet.
4. *Emotional First Signs*. Jane felt a rush of upsetting emotions that were set off by the phone call with her mother. These included feelings of anger, guilt, and sadness. These feelings (a) motivated her to seek something fast to soothe her and, (b) drew her to an unhealthy choice.
5. *Behavioral First Signs*. As she walked through the living room, she stopped and looked at the cake for a long time. She also took steps towards it and eventually picked it up.

After looking over the following two Info Boxes, you can turn to the next Skill Boxes. These will train you in how to identify Triggers.

INFO BOX #13 -
Sample Triggers that Increase Pain Flares

- Obsessing on Anxious Thoughts
- Lack of Sleep
- Re-Focusing on Bad Memories or the Pain
- Imagining a Painful Future
- Impatient Feelings
- Multi-Tasking
- Annoying People
- Unhealthy Foods
- Intense Stimulation (i.e., Loud Noises)
- Extreme Work or Activity Load
- Arguments

INFO BOX #14 -
Sample First Signs that Warn You about a Pain Flare

- Confusion, Overwhelm and Sadness
- Worry and Anxiety
- Muscle Tension
- Fast Heart Beats
- Boredom
- Sleeplessness and Fatigue
- Feelings of Hopelessness and Helplessness
- Loneliness

Skills of the Day - Noticing Negatives

(A)
"Revealing Triggers"

The Skill Box below describes one method you can use to identify a Trigger. It shows you how to "look backward" by thinking about the pain or upsetting episodes that have happened in the past, and recalling what may have set them off.

NOTICING SKILL BOX #1 -
"Revealing Triggers"

Step One- Revealing Triggers. After a pain flare passes, think back to what was going on the previous day or two before the flare hit you. Identify the Triggers in your Physical, Social, and Activity Worlds that may have set it off. Here are some useful questions:

A) *Physical Triggers.* Ask yourself:
- "What was the weather like?"
- "Did I have a cold, flu, or other illness?"
- "Were there loud sounds or intense smells that irritated me?"

B) *Social Triggers.* Ask yourself:
- "Did anyone annoy me before the flare?"
- "Did I hear some bad news regarding someone I care about?"
- "Did a friend or family member just criticize me?"

C) *Activity Triggers.* Ask yourself:
- "What activities did I do before the flare came?"
- "How many strenuous activities did I do?"
- "Did I get stressed out while doing something today?"

D) *Other Triggers.* "Did I get an unexpected bill on the mail?"

Step Two - Make a Trigger List. Using a journal or digital file, record the Triggers that you identified.

Step Three - Watch Out for "Repeaters." Once you've made your list, notice any Triggers that happen a lot. Each time you notice this, pull out your list and place a check mark after this repeating Trigger. This Step can better help you to catch and disarm that Trigger.

Step Four - Add to the List. Over the weeks and months, add to the List new Triggers and Repeaters that you discover and keep a copy with you.

Step Five – Using Your Trigger List. The list will alert you to the Triggers that pop up and remind you to disarm them by using some of the other Comfort Skills. In this way, you can better control your relationship with pain. For example, if arguing with your spouse is a Trigger, you can 1) stop the argument, 2) use the "Breath Count" Skill to calm your nervous system, and 3) do something fun to raise your mood.

(B)
"Revealing First Signs"

Another Negative to notice is a "First Sign," which is a reaction in your mind and/or body to a Trigger.

NOTICING SKILL BOX #2 -
"Revealing First Signs"

Step One - Look Backwards - What Happened Before the Episode. Choose a stressful incident or pain flare that recently happened. Sit comfortably and recall what happened over the previous 12-to-24-hours in your body and mind before the flare hit.

Step Two - Finding First Signs. Recall any physical sensations, thoughts, imaginings, emotions, or behaviors that you noticed. You can use these questions to identify First Signs:

- *Physical First Sign.* Ask yourself, "Were there any tensions or unusual sensations in my body before the flare hit?" If so, then ask, "Where did you feel it in my body?" Example - A tight neck comes before a headache.

Step Three - Make a First Sign List. Using your journal or digital file, record any First Signs you discovered.

Step Four - Watch for "Repeaters." Once you've made your list, notice any First Signs that happen a lot. Put a check next to them.

Step Five - Add to the List. Over the comings weeks and months, add to your list whenever you notice new First Signs or Repeaters. Keep it with you.

Step Six – Using Your First Sign List. As you notice these First Signs popping up in the future, draw from the other Comfort Strategies to better control your relationship with pain. Example – If you notice that the chronic pain tends to increase after you feel fatigued (Physical First Sign), then you might take evasive action by 1) resting, 2) listening to some soothing music, and/or 3) using a Re-Focusing Skill for 20 to 30 minutes (i.e., Meditation).

STORY BOX #11 - Jack the Salesman

Jack is a 40-year-old used car salesman who survived a skiing accident that left him with chronic left shoulder pain. About halfway through his work day, he'd get a 9/10 pain level that drives him crazy. Typically, in the middle of a sales pitch, he'd have to excuse himself because of the throbbing pain in his arm. When this happened, he had to lie down and take a pill for the breakthrough pain. This often put him to sleep, which would ruin the rest of his sales day and make him feel miserable. Jack eventually learned how to use the "Revealing First Sign" Skill. He soon noticed that one frequent First Sign of a potential pain flare was a tight feeling in his neck. Other times, he observed that the flare would come after he worried a lot about a particular sale. He used these First Signs to remind himself to stop what he was doing and practice the "Breath Massage" Skill. This shortened the pain flares and often allowed him to return to work.

STORY BOX #12 - Medicine Worry

Alyce is a retired nurse who suffers from nearly constant leg pain. She was using a number of heavy-duty pain medications that took a long time to bring her only a little relief. Using the "Revealing First Sign" Skill, she recalled that when she took a dose of medication, this would set off a worry thought such as, "When will the damn pills start working!" This was soon followed by another First Sign - increased anxiety – which intensified the chronic pain and convinced Alyce to over-use her medication. After seeing this pattern clearly, she started taking evasive action whenever these Signs showed themselves. She would (a) raise her mood with an Enjoying Skill (Laughter), and (b) practice a Re-Focusing Skill ("Breath Massage"). After using these Strategies, Alyce discovered that her Comfort level rose faster than it took for the medication to work! From that day on, she was always on the lookout for worry thoughts and anxious feelings and committed herself to transforming them with her Comfort Skills.

The Last Practice
"Breath Massage"

How would you like to have a massage whenever you desired one? You can when you imagine moving your breath in and out of various parts of your body. Pain, low moods, and stress usually make your body feel very tense. This next Re-Focusing Skill helps you to release that tension by allowing you to calmly drift into a very deep state of relaxation. Using the instructions in the next Box, you'll feel as if each breath is massaging and soothing your body.

RE-FOCUSING SKILL BOX #2 –
"Breath Massage"

Step One – Sit, Set a Timer, and Settle In. First, find a quiet place to sit and set a timer for five minutes. (Over time, build this up to twenty-minutes a session.) Choose a seat or recliner that will comfortably support your body. Remember, if you lie down, you may fall asleep.

Step Two – Three Deep Breaths in the Belly. Start by taking three deep breaths in and out of your belly and focus on the feeling of your belly moving out and in with each breath. (If the belly is an uncomfortable place to focus, imagine feeling the breath move in another part of your body (i.e., hands).

Step Three - Initial Body Focus. Next, allow the breath to continue on its own as you direct your attention to one part of your body (i.e., fingers, toes). Notice how that body parts feel - Warm or cool? Light or heavy? Soft or solid? Another sensation? Concentrate on this for a moment.

Step Four - Breath Massage. Now, imagine that your breaths move in and out of that part of the body, massaging it with each inhale and exhale. You can imagine something visual (i.e., colors flowing through the body part).

Step Five - Move to the Next Part. After five to ten breaths, take a slow, deep breath into that body part and, as you breathe out, let it fade, float, or drift away. Pause for a few seconds, then imagine the breath flowing in and out of the next body part, soothing and massaging it (see Body Parts Box below). Continue this step until you have gone through most or all of your whole body. ***Remember***, you can skip uncomfortable parts & move to those that feel better.

Step Six - Full Body Breath Massage. After you've relaxed all your body parts, let the breath massage your entire body. Take in a deep breath and imagine a light or good feeling entering the bottoms of your feet and going up your body 'till it reaches your belly. As you exhale, imagine this good feeling flows through your upper body and arms and exits out the top of your head. Give yourself this "full body massage" for as many breaths as you'd like.

Step Seven - Returning. When you're ready to finish this practice session, take three slow, deep breaths and, as you exhale for the third time, allow your eyes to slowly open, refreshed, calm, and alert.

Remember

- **"Just Do It to Do It**." Free yourself from having to make or seek any particular results. "Just do it to do it and notice what happens." Don't force the relaxation, just allow the Comfort to come in its own time.

- **Choosing Body Parts**. Skip any body parts that hurt too much and direct your attention to those that are more comfortable (i.e., if hands hurt, focus on your forearms or elbows). See Body Parts Box for suggested order.

- **Let Go of Unwanted Distractions and Return to Focus**. When a distracting thought, memory, image, feeling, sound, or anything tries to move your awareness away from the breath, let go of it and return your attention back to focus.

Okay, now use his Skill and sit for at least ten minutes and practice massaging your body with your breath.

INFO BOX #17 -
"Body Parts to Relax"

➢ *Toes*
➢ *Bottom of feet and heels*
➢ *Top of feet and ankles*
➢ *Lower legs*
➢ *Knees*
➢ *Thighs into hips, bottom, and pelvis*
➢ *Belly and lower back*
➢ *Chest and upper back*
➢ *Hands and wrists*
➢ *Forearms into the elbows*
➢ *Upper arm over the shoulders*
➢ *Neck*
➢ *Back, sides, and top of head*
➢ *Face*

HOMEWORK BOX
FIRST TRAINING DAY – WEEK 2

1. **Breath Massage.** Use the Re-Focusing Skill above to practice 10-to-20-minutes at least once each day.

2. **Identify Triggers and First Signs.** Use the Noticing Skills Boxes on pages 148 and 149 to identify three Triggers that set off flares or upsetting situations, and three First Signs that come before a pain flare or emotional upset.

3. **Continue to Develop and Pursue Your Goals**.

Noticing Positives and Laughing Your Head Off
Second Training Day – Week 2

The Skill Review

"Breath Massage"
Take at least 15 minutes to massage your body with your breath (see page 152).

Today's Pain Problems
Pain Problem #2 – "Attention Hijacked by Pain and Stress"
Pain Problem #4 – "Sadness, Worry, and Other Miserable Feelings"
Pain Problem #8 – "Missing the Good Things in Your Life"

Learn/About #6 –
The Enjoying Strategy & Enjoying Right Now

"Enjoying Strategy" *is the practice of raising your mood, positively coping with upsetting situations, and strengthening your positive qualities and sense of personal meaning.* The basic definition of the word "enjoy" is to "rejoice and be glad." It's also derived from the Old French word *"enjoir,"* which means "to give joy" or "to take delight in." It also means to "take pleasure in." If we look at the word more closely, we'll see that it's made up of two parts: 1) **En**, which means "to make," and 2) **Joy,** which describes "pleasure or delight."[46] Together, these define "Enjoying" as an active practice, one that requires you to put in the time, effort, and energy that is necessary to create pleasure. When you engage in Enjoying Skills, you're purposely doing things to "take delight" and "make joy." The challenge is to do this even when you're not feel very joyful.

Here's the happy truth: When you pursue pleasure and happiness, pain and Misery tend to partially (or sometimes fully) fade away. Sounds too simple, right?! It's very difficult to get yourself to do pleasurable things when you're hurting or feeling depressed, anxious, or angry. When you're feeling bad, advice such as "Follow Your Bliss" or "Seek Enjoyment" or "Don't Worry, Be Happy" sounds like namby-pamby, FuFu self-help Kaka. On the other hand, about twenty years of scientific research finds that when you purposely engage in joyful practices and cultivate positive thoughts and attitudes, you'll experience a good feeling that grows and expands.[47] In addition, you may also become more creative, productive, social, and healthy. Most importantly.

---

[46] See Online Etymology Dictionary. You can find it online at Etymonline.com.
[47] See "Positivity" by Barbara Fredrickson (2009).

What is most important to you, you'll feel better. As you respond happily to pleasurable experiences, your brain will increase your Comfort level, which enables your nervous system to reduce its sensitivity to pain. For example, when you're "Enjoying Right Now," you'll engage in fun and laughter right now! The more you do that, the easier you'll feel. (See page 94-95 for a brief discussion on one source of Enjoying: Positive Psychology.)

Learn/About #7 –Four Health Effects of Laughter

When you laugh (and even smile), your Comfort level improves.[48] This is caused by four factors. **First**, pain relief is enhanced by an increase in your Endorphin levels. This is one of your body's "feel good" hormones. (It actually stands for "Endogenous Morphine.") Endorphins act like a natural pain medication, numbing some of the effects of the pain process (and they cause no bad side effects).[49] Your body produces them when you laugh, exercise, or get happily excited. A **second** benefit of laughter is that it provides you with a positive distraction, which reduces pain perception and the hypersensitivity in your brain.[50] **Third**, it reduces stress hormones, which typically strain your physiology and worsen pain sensations. With less stress hormones irritating your system, your body will feel more at ease.[51] The **fourth** effect of laughter is that it raises your mood to a happier place. Distressing emotional states, like depression and anxiety, make you vulnerable to painful sensations. Positive emotions, like joy, have the opposite effect, desensitizing your body to pain signals. These and other positive effects of laughter are listed in the Laughter Info Box below.[52]

Laugh When You're Sad

Unbelievable! – How can I suggest that you start to giggle in the middle of your Misery? Obviously, when you feel bad, you're usually not in the mood to laugh. Yet, studies on humor have shown that ***your brain does not know the difference between real and fake laughter!*** [53] That's right – when you squeeze out a bunch of "ha, ha's," even when you're not happy, your brain will respond as if you were really laughing and that lead to benefits (see below). The intentional practice of laughing is even promoted by an international laughter

---

[48] http://www.webmd.com/balance/video/laughter-benefits
[49] https://simple.wikipedia.org/wiki/Endorphins
[50] http://www.huffingtonpost.com/2011/09/15/laughter-pain-tolerance_n_962353.html
[51] http://www.bodyinmind.org/stress-model-of-chronic-pain-vachon-presseau/
[52] "Anticipating a Laugh Reduces Our Stress Hormones," in American Psychological Society (April, 2008); "Modulation of Neuroimmune Parameters During the Eustress of Humor-Associated Mirthful Laughter," by Lee Berk and colleagues in Alternative Therapies in Health and Medicine (March 2001).
[53] See "The Best Medicine" by Joe Hoare in *Nursing Standard*, Volume 19 (Issue 16), pages 18-19, and https://www.researchgate.net/profile/Michel_Woodbury/publication/286522472_Laughter_Yoga_Benefits_of_Mixing_Laughter_and_Yoga/links/578efd2708ae35e97c3f7b15.pdf

club that purposely encourages participants to playfully pretend to laugh until they start doing it for real.[54]

LAUGHTER FACT BOX -
Positive Effects from Laughter

Health Benefits
- Reduces pain and suffering
- Reduces depression
- Reduces stress and tension
- Lowers blood pressure
- Increases relaxation (after the laughing has calmed)
- Strengthens heart function
- Improves your circulation
- Increases muscle flexibility
- Increases the oxygen in your body by boosting the respiratory system
- Boosts your immunity by increasing infection-fighting cells and proteins
- Produces a general sense of well-being

Other Positive Effects
- Provides you a "muscle workout" and may reduce calories (when you laugh one hundred times/day)
- Increases social connections
- Distracts you from negative emotions and sensations
- Enhances your optimism about your life

---

[54] http://www.laughteryoga.org/

STORY BOX #13 –
Caroline's Laughing Fit

Caroline is a young woman suffering from terrible migraine headaches. Often in the Workshop, I'd see her sitting with her head down. However, one day she gave all of us a pleasant surprise when she told this story:

"I was visiting my mom and little sister the other day and we were sitting at the kitchen table talking. After a while, my head started hurting and I began thinking that I'd have to leave soon to get to bed before the migraine flare hit her full on. Having to leave made my headache worse because I get frustrated over not having a life. I mean, hell, I couldn't stay and do something as normal as hang out with my family.

"Just as I was getting ready to excuse myself, my sister said something very funny and my mom and I began to chuckle a little. Then things got worse – my sister reacted by laughing really hard, so hard that she fell off of her chair! This set my mom off and she began howling like a hyena! I began to laugh uncontrollably and my entire body shook up a storm. Then, when I tried to help my sister up, I ended up on the floor with her. For the next twenty minutes, the three of us were shrieking our heads off in laughter – my mom holding on to the table and my sister and I rolling around on the floor. When it was all over, the headache was down to a 2/10. I stayed with them for the rest of the day and we giggled on and off each time one of use recalled our laughing spree."

Skills of the Day

(A)
"Laughing"

The next two Enjoying Skill Boxes suggest a number of ways you can practice "Laughing" on a regular basis.

ENGOYING SKILL BOX #1 –
"Laughing"

Short-Term Laughs

1. **Watch Something Funny.** This can include watching movies, plays, TV shows, kids at play, or comedy on YouTube (see the "Funny Box" later in this Training Day section).

2. **Jokes.** Read jokes and tell them to a friend (or to your pet).

3. **Funny Moment Replay.** Recall a funny moment in your life and relive it again in your imagination. Tell your story to a friend.

4. **Get Close to Group Laughter.** Sometimes at a party or other social gathering, you'll hear laughter coming from a small group of people. If the situation is safe, draw close to the group and breathe in the laughter like fresh air. People usually enjoy sharing funny moments, so you might not be intruding when you come over and listen.

5. **Invite Humor.** When you're talking with people you know, ask them if they'd like to exchange funny stories or jokes.

Long-Term Laughs

1. **The Daily Laugh.** Do something to get yourself to laugh for at least ten to thirty minutes every day. Given the incredible health effects that come from laughter, a "daily dose" will help you like a soothing tonic.

2. **Hang Out with Playful People.** These are people who laugh easily at themselves and at life's absurdities. They often found humor in everyday events. You'll discover that their playful points of view and laughter are contagious.

3. **Attend a Laughter Yoga Club.** This international movement encourages people to laugh. It was founded in 1995 by a physician from India named Madan Kataria. Over the years, it has grown to over 6000 Laughter Yoga clubs located in sixty-eight countries (as of 2013). Club sessions are free. They usually meet for thirty-minutes and include laughing and breathing exercises and a little quiet meditation at the end. You may find this an enjoyable way to laugh in a safe environment. Find a local club by searching online at LaughterYoga.org, and see their videos on YouTube.

4. **Attend an Improvisational Comedy Class or Theater Group or Go to a Comedy Club.** If you want to put more time and effort into developing your sense of humor and have a lot of fun, join a comedy class or theater group. At a minimum, the other students will make you laugh. You can also regularly attend a local comedy club and get some laughs there.

WARNING!! ➔ Please make sure to avoid vigorous belly laughs if they exacerbate the pain

STORY BOX #14 –
Grumpy to Happy

Harvey used to have a sense of humor. However, after his work accident, he lost the full use of his right arm because it throbbed and burned, making him feel incredibly miserable and depressed. For the first six sessions of the Comfort Workshop, he didn't smile, even when he reported having an easier week. In fact, he once sadly reported that his five-year-old daughter began calling him "Grumpy" after she saw the Disney cartoon "*Snow White and the Seven Dwarves.*"

Things began to turn around for Harvey after he decided to do the Daily Laugh assignment. He watched the Comedy Channel on Cable TV every day and in a short period of time (like right away), he'd clock in about an hour of laughter each day. Later in the Workshop, Harvey would tell us joke after joke until we had to either shut him up or get laughed out of our chairs! He was extremely funny and he added a lot to our group. As a result of his humor, he began to feel and sleep better. Because he could function more comfortably, he decided to attend a comedy class at a local performance arts school. After some time, his daughter stopped calling him Grumpy and, instead, renamed him "Happy."

BONUS
The Funny Box

Laughter often comes more easily when you watch something funny. If you can stop what you're doing right now, go to your computer, and watch a funny something for at least 20 minutes on YouTube – maybe you'll choose to see some of the following comedy videos.

FUNNY BOX
Suggested Comedy Video Titles on YouTube
Comedy for All Ages

1. **Bill Cosby.**
   - Bill Cosby – Dentists
   - Bill Cosby – Grandparents
   - Bill Cosby – Himself Stand Up Show
2. **Stephan Colbert.**
   - Whose Line is it Anyway – Scene to rap with Stephen Colbert
   - Stephen Colbert on the O'Reilly Factor
3. **Gilda Radner.**
   - Society of Stupid People
4. **Jon Stewart.**
   - William Kristol talks with Jon Stewart
5. **Carol Burnett.**
   - Carol Burnett show Outtakes – Tim Conway's Elephant Story
6. **I Love Lucy.**
   - Lucy's Famous Chocolate Scene

Adult Comedy

1. **Whose Line is it Anyway?**
   - Whose Line is it Anyway - Questions Only (Whoopie Goldberg)
   - Whose Line is it Anyway – Richard Simmons (Hilarious!)
   - Whose Line is it Anyway? Robin Williams
   - Whose Line: Newsflash – the Beast!!
2. **Pablo Francisco**.
   - Pablo Francisco Movie Guy
   - Pablo Francisco - White Guy insulting Mexicans
3. **Russell Peters**.
   - Russel Peters: Cheap Jews, Indians, and Chinese
4. **George Carlin.**
   - George Carlin Talks about "Stuff"
   - George Carlin – 7 Words **(Warning – this is very profane!)**
   - George Carlin – George's Best Stuff

---

5. **Whoopie Goldberg**.
   - Whoopie Goldberg's opening monologue at the 71st Academy Awards
   - Whoopie Goldberg – Direct from Broadway 1985
6. **Eddie Murphy**.
   - Eddie Murphy – Delirious Full
7. **Chris Tucker**.
   - Chris Tucker – Random 93 Jokes
8. **George Lopez**.
   - George Lopez - Why You Crying Part 1
9. **Rich Little**.
   - Rich Little – Comedian Impressionist
10. **Don Rickles**.
    - Don Rickles on Dean Martin Roasts Bob Hope
11. **Robin Williams**.
    - Robin Williams: Inside the Actors Studio Part 1
    - Stand Up Comedy: Robin Williams on Broadway

Final Note – Even When You Smile

Researchers have also found that merely smiling can lift your mood. When you make a "Big Smile," one where you lift the sides of your mouth up and squint your eyes a little, your body releases mood-raising hormones and neurotransmitters such as serotonin and dopamine.[55]

Some scientists suggest that smiling also creates other positive health effects.[56] Even if you smile when you're not feeling happy, you can receive these benefits. In other words, your brain cannot tell the difference between real and fake smiles.

(B)
"Doing Fun"

For some of you, life isn't as fun as it used to be. Perhaps you've given up on seeking the things that once gave you pleasure. True, there are some activities you can no longer do comfortably, but there are plenty of new doable ones out there waiting for you to discover. You might also find that you're able to return to old pleasures by doing them in a different

---

[55] Hess, U. & Blairy, S. (2001). Facial mimicry and emotional contagion to dynamic emotional facial expressions and their influence on decoding accuracy. International Journal of Psychophysiology. 40, 129-141.
[56] Abel, MH, Hester, R. (2002). The therapeutic effects of smiling, in An empirical reflection on the smile. Mellen studies in psychology, Vol. 4. (pp. 217-253). Lewiston, NY, US: Edwin Mellen Press; Surakka, V., & Hietanen. Also J. K. (1998). Facial and emotional reactions to Duchenne and non-Duchenne smiles. International Journal of Psychophysiology.29, 23–33.

way (i.e., walking fifteen minutes in a park instead of trekking five miles up a mountain trail). Like other Skills, when you practice "Doing Fun," it's like building a muscle – the more you exercise it, the stronger you get. The following Skill Box offers one way to return to Fun.

ENJOYING SKILL BOX #2 - "Doing Fun"

Building a Fun Menu. Here is one way to discover and collect enjoyable activities:

- *Step One - Get Ready.* Sit down comfortably with pen and paper, a journal, or digital file.

- *Step Two - Recall.* Close your eyes, let your mind roam through your memory and recall
  - ➤ What you used to enjoy doing?
  - ➤ What you think you might enjoy doing now?
  - ➤ What enjoyable activities have you been doing lately?

- *Step Three – Make a List of these Activities.* Write whatever activities come to mind and don't cut any out.

- *Step Four – Separate Out Painful Activities.* Identify those activities on the list that are usually pretty painful and turn them into a "Do it Differently" Menu. Later, you can use the "Do it Differently" bonus section below to return to some form of these activities.

- *Step Five – Order the Fun Menu.* The activities that remain on your original list will comprise your "Fun Menu." Now, put them into order from "most desired to least desired" fun activity. (IE, 1-Going to a movie, 2-taking a walk, 3-shopping for clothes, etc.)

- *Step Six – Try it On!* Pick an activity from the list and decide how you'll do it -- Then, do it! Remember, you don't have to do a lot.

- *Step Seven - Evaluate.* Soon after you finish the activity, think about it. Did you have fun? What worked; what didn't? Would you like to do it again, add to it, or put it away and do something different?

- *Step Eight - Do Another One.* Repeat Steps Five through Seven as many times as you'd like.

Fun Menu Types. Once you've identified and tried out several enjoyable things to do, you can create a couple of "menus" that include some of your favorite activities.

  A) *The "Quick Fun" Menu.* This is made up of activities you can plan and do within an hour or so. Example – Perhaps you'll decide to go to a café and read a book, go for a walk, call a friend, take in a movie, or eat a nice meal at a local restaurant.

  B) *The "Big Fun" Menu.* This Menu has activities that'll take some time to prepare for and carry out (and they're well worth it). Example –Taking a short trip with a friend or a sweetheart to a Bed-and-Breakfast hotel for a week-end, or attending a music festival or ball game.

BONUS – "Do it Differently"

Intro – Pain and Misery like to tell you that you "can't do anything anymore!" Good thing they're wrong – you may be able to engage in a number of activities you used to do. The question is → how can you do them differently.

Pick One and Tweak It – Using the "Do it Differently" Menu you created in the previous Skill Box, choose an activity and plan how to do a small part of it, or carry it out in a new way that makes it very doable & relatively comfortable.

Mini-Story – Cynthia loved cooking and would do a lot of it before her back went out. Now, she had to stop because she could not stand very long and could not lift heavy pots full of food without a pain flare. She eventually decided to "Do it Differently" and restructured cooking to fit her body. What did that look like? – first, she figured out that she could do a number of cooking activities while sitting (which was better). She'd also put an empty pot on the stove, fill it and then get her family members to move it around when the time came. If she wanted to cook, a big meal she'd do small tasks (i.e., cut vegetables) over several days before the meal. As she got close to the time she's invite over a person or two to help her with larger cooking tasks. Clean-up, of course, fell on other family members and willing friends. In this way, Cynthia did it differently and was able to return to hosting dinner parties (see another Do It Differently story on page 167).

(C)
"I Want to See More of…"

"Positives" *are satisfying changes and events that increase your comfort and well-being*. You might wonder how you can experience Positives when pain tends to take up much of your day. Because of the human tendency to focus on upsetting and disappointing things that come our way, it's normal to miss the good things that come along.

There are two sets of questions that help you notice Positives in your life and discover what caused them. Although it may be challenging to answer these questions, as you do you'll make some surprising discoveries. [57]

The first of these is found in the "I Want to See More of…." Skill Box. It shows you how to notice what's going well by directing you to track the Positives that presently arise in your life (even small ones). Scientists have found that when you purposely notice and immerse yourself in good memories or pleasurable activities, your Comfort level rises.[58]

The following Noticing Skill Box, and an accompanying Story Box, will describe the first question and how you can use it. [59]

NOTICING SKILL BOX # 3 - "I Want to See More of…"

The Questions. The two questions below direct you to observe good things that are going on in your daily life and to help you to discover what makes them happen. Positive events may not show up a lot, or look very big, but they are there. Even small changes in any part of your life are good and they grow as you notice them.

- "What's Been Happening Lately, Large or Small, That I Want to See More of in My Life?"
- "What Caused These Things to Happen?"

Record what you discovered in your journal or digital file.

Not "Wishful Thinking"

This is not asking, "What do I wish was going on?" – that's a different question. Instead, it invites you to notice what is already going on in your life now that brings you even a little happiness.

---

[57] This idea is adapted from concepts and practices developed by the creators of Solution-Focused therapy. See "Handbook of Solution-Focused Brief Therapy," by Scott Miller.

[58] "The How of Happiness: A New Approach to Getting the Life You Want" by Sonja Lyubomirsky

[59] In Week Eight you'll learn the second set of Positive questions looking at how your situation has improved.

STORY BOX #15 –
Ruthie's Amazing Story

Ruthie is a 45-year-old accountant who was very consumed by chronic pain and felt frustrated about the limits that it placed on her. Week after week, she'd sit in the Comfort Skills Workshop and report no improvement in her life, while most members of the class described a variety of changes.

Ruthie talked about what was going badly, such as the severe neuropathic pain in her feet. She also worried about her ability to concentrate and to recall things. This caused her to make a number of mistakes in her payroll accounts and her supervisor was starting to put pressure on her to "get it together." After twenty years working as a successful accountant, this problem left her feeling very bad about herself.

During one particular session, I asked everyone to go around and answer this question → "What's been happening lately - large or small - that you want to see more of in your life?" To the group's surprise, Ruthie spoke up and said:

"A month ago, out of desperation, I decided to practice 20 minutes of Mantra/Breath Meditation every morning before going to work. Sometimes I did it for a few minutes on my breaks. I recently noticed that I was making fewer mistakes in my work, and that my boss stopped bugging me about it. I feel a whole lot better going to my job now."

Since then, Ruthie has practiced meditation regularly and continues to enjoy a considerable improvement in her concentration, job performance, and Comfort level.

Okay, now think about the last few weeks and ask yourself, *"What's been happening lately, large or small, that I want to see more of in my life?"* At first, this might be a bit challenging to do. That's fine, take your time and keep trying – you'll discover something fairly soon. Once you do, write it down in a journal or digital file.

STORY BOX #16 –
Paula Does It Differently at the Movies

I once worked with Paula, a lovely 36-year-old mother of three who suffered terribly from Arachnoiditis, a very painful spinal condition. She was very depressed when she first came to see me and would painfully get up and down off the recliner chair in my office as we talked. She could only sit for fifteen minutes at a time.

Paula told me that she loved to go to the movies but felt conflicted because her disability prevented her from sitting long. She also admitted that when she did go, she felt very embarrassed each time she had to get up and down in front of all of the theater goers to relieve the stress on her back. In her mind, the only way she could attend a movie theater was the way that her Old Body had done it, sitting still through a two-hour film in a crowded theater.

I asked her if she ever thought of doing it differently? This was difficult for her because she focused a great deal on her Old Body (the one without much pain). However, in time, she was able to accept that she had a New Body (one sensitive to pain) and this motivated her to create a New Normal in her life.

Her first step was to go to the movies in a new way. She first arranged an early afternoon ride to the theater that would take her there in the middle of the week when there were few people going to the show. She chose a movie house that had the "cool" recliner chairs for disabled folks. On the day she went, Paula found that she could pace her sitting time by getting up and down every fifteen or twenty minutes. By going alone (and later with friends and family), she cut down on her embarrassment. The first time she did this, it worked so well that she stayed for <u>two</u> movies, had a great time, and on that day, she wasn't bothered by depression or a pain flare. By doing what she loved in a different manner, Paula was able to return to some of the pleasures she had in her Old Body.

The Last Practice
"Breath Massage"

Take at least 15 minutes to massage your body with your breath (see page 152).

HOMEWORK BOX
SECOND TRAINING DAY – WEEK 2

1. **Breath Massage.** Practice the Breath Massage at least once each day or night. See if you can increase your practice over time (see page 152).

2. **Laugh Your Head Off for Thirty Minutes a Day!** Use your own resources, the Skill Boxes, and the "Funny Box" above to laugh 30 minutes each day.

3. **Start Noticing Positive Change.** In the days between training sessions, notice any large or small, positive changes in your life. At first, these may be very small. At the end of each day, ask yourself the following, then write down your answer:

"What happened today, large or small, that I want to see more of in my life?"

The Comfort Account in Your Body Bank
Third Training Day – Week 2

The Skill Review

(A)
"Breath Massage"

By now, you might discover that this Skill is becoming easier to do and may lead to more relaxation. Practice it for 20 minutes right now (see page 152).

(B)
"I Want to See More of..."

Consult your journal or digital file, and answer the two questions below.

- **"What happened since the last Training Day, large or small, that I want to see more of in my life?"**
- **"What caused these things to happen?"**

Today's Pain Problem
Pain Problem #11 – "Unbalanced Activity"

Learn/About #8 –
The Comfort Account in Your "Body Bank"

It's common for many of you keep some of your money in a checking account at your bank. You probably know what would happen if you wrote checks that exceeded the amount of money you have in your account — you'd get overdrawn or go bankrupt! This fact motivates most people to use their account carefully.

You can apply this money management approach to your activity life by imagining that your body is like a bank. Instead of money, your **"Body Bank"** contains a **"Comfort Account"** filled with **"Comfort Time,"** *which is the amount of time and energy that you can spend doing activities comfortably.* The more time and effort you spend on activities that are physically and emotionally taxing, the faster you use up your Comfort Time.

"Recovery Time" *is the amount of time you spend taking a break from activities that stress your pain condition.* When you take breaks, you can build up your Comfort Account and this allows you to return to activities feeling refreshed and more comfortable. If you don't take some Recovery Time (i.e., by resting), you'll use up all of your Comfort Time and that can lead to increased pain flares.

You have to be careful in choosing what activities you do because some may be "more expensive" than others. For example, let's say that you want to exercise and you have a painful shoulder. On the one hand, if you do push-ups, you quickly discover that that activity is "too expensive" for your body because it causes a pain flare. On the other hand, if you do gentle stretching and strengthening, you won't lose all of your Comfort Time and your body will feel better.

Skills of the Day

(A)
"Pay As You Go – Three Options"

One way to carefully spend your Comfort Time is by using the "Pay As You Go" Skill. Healthcare professionals call this "activity pacing," and it's similar to how you responsibly pay your bills. For example, when you don't have enough money to cover all your bills at once, you might pace your spending by paying off some bills now and others later. In other words, you allow your checkbook to "rest" until you have earned enough money to pay your remaining debts. You can apply this practice to your body by restructuring your activity so that you conserve some of your energy and effort and reduce stress and pain. By doing this, you prevent yourself from "overdrawing" on your Comfort Account, and this reduces the risk of a pain flare. Following the next story, you'll learn three "Pay As You Go Options."

STORY BOX #17 – Janet's Laundry

Janet suffers from Fibromyalgia, a disease that originates in the Central Nervous System, causing pain in her muscles and joints. Because she is often flared after doing chores, she decided to apply a "Pay As You Go" option to her weekly laundry task. First, Janet used a Noticing Skill ("Revealing Triggers") and observed that soon after washing, drying, folding, and putting away her three loads of laundry on a typical Sunday, she'd experience the "Mother of All Flares" on Monday, Tuesday, and Wednesday. This forced her into a bed of excruciating pain.

Next, she decided to avoid this kind of flare by doing only one load of laundry <u>every other day</u>. Finally, she saved her body's Comfort Time by only working on low-impact tasks during the interim days (i.e., washing a few dishes), and taking some Recovery Time to rest. When she looked back some weeks later, she noticed that this one change reduced her flare-ups by 50% and increased her ability to do other things she desired.

MOVING SKILL BOX #2 –
"Pay As You Go – Three Options"

Option One – "The Do Lists"

These help you prioritize tasks, allowing you to do the most important ones first, the next important next, and so on.

Setting Up the Lists.

- *Step One – the Journal.* Set up a page in a journal or digital file to organize your lists.

- *Step Two – Brain Storming.* Sit comfortably and write down all the errands, tasks, and activities you want to complete in a week, even if they sound too big. This is your "Brainstorm List."

- *Step Three – Build the "A-List."* Go through the Brain-Storming List, pick out the most important and doable items, and put them on a separate page labeled, *"A-List."* These are tasks that you need to get done as soon as possible. Sort these tasks in order of priority (i.e., most to least important).

- *Step Four – Order the "A List."* Organize the items on this list in order of priority (i.e., a- Do laundry, b- Do dishes, c- call the Plummer, etc).

- *Step Five – Build the "B List."* Look at what is left on your Do List and pick out items that you consider moderately important. Write these on a *"B-List"* page. These are tasks that you desire to finish over the next two-to-three weeks. Just as you did for the A-List, prioritize these.

- *Step Six – Order the "B List."* Organize the items on this list in order of priority (i.e., a- Do laundry, b- Do dishes, c- call the Plummer, etc).

Using the Lists.

- *Step One – Begin Doing the Tasks on the "A List".* On the first day, carry out the tasks at the top of your A-List. These might include "do two loads of laundry, shop for a microwave, call my mother, etc." As you complete a task, cross it out.

- *Step Two - Pace yourself.* Take several breaks throughout the day.

- *Step Three – Time to Stop.* <u>The most important step</u> → As the day wears on, you'll notice a number of items still left on your list. You'll also become aware that the day is running out and so is your energy and Comfort level. At that point, *stop for the day*. Notice the items left on your A-List and plan to do some of them tomorrow or the day after.

- *Step Four.* The next work day, repeat Steps One through Three. Do the same each day until you've completed your A-List. Once you finish those tasks, start on your B-List.

- *Step Five.* At the end of the week, set up a new list for the next week using any leftover and new tasks. (See the Margie'sExample Box below.)

Option Two – "Time Over Task"

The Zeigarnik Effect. Most people in our culture are taught to focus on tasks and work on them until they are completed (i.e., clean the whole house). A psychological phenomenon discovered over ninety years ago by a Russian scientist is the "Zeigarnik Effect." It's our tendency to continually think about an unfinished task until we complete it.

The Problem. So here it is → Because we tend to over-focus on a task until it's finished, we may become tempted to Over-Do some of our chores until we end up with a pain flare.

Practice the Solution. "Time Over Task." In order to better deal with the pain flares caused by Over-Doing, you can change your expectations about activities. *Instead of thinking "task," think "time" or "amount."* Before engaging in an errand, a chore, or another demanding activity, ask yourself this question:

"How much time can I spend doing this activity and still feel comfortable afterwards?"

"Time & Amount" - Examples.

- *Example One – "Thinking Time."* Let's say that you are about to do the dishes. Replace the thought, "I have to keep washing the dishes until they're all done," with the idea, "I will do the dishes for ten-minutes and then I'll take a break." You might do this one or more rounds and then stop completely for a long break.

- *Example Two – "Thinking Amount."* In some situations, you can focus on amount. Instead of thinking about doing "all of the dishes," you might think to yourself, "I'll do a third of the dishes now and another third in a couple of hours." There are times when that's too much and you decide to wait for the next day to do clean more dishes.

Option Three – "Activity Balancing"

You might find yourself spending too much time engaged on one activity. This Skill encourages you to balance the following three activities:

A. **Pain Stressing Activity.** Any action you take that strains you physically and/or emotionally and will lead to more pain (i.e., gardening for hours).

B. **Pain Neutral Activity**. This activity does not provide you much relief, but neither does it make things worse. It may include short breaks or movements that won't exacerbate the pain (i.e., a short walk for someone with Fibromyalgia).

C. **Pain Relieving Activity**. This includes activities that raise your comfort level (i.e., watching a movie, laughing).

Balancing Activities – An Example. One fellow suffered from arm pain caused by a repetitive stress injury. One day he got fed up with the pile of dishes in his sink and decided to wash them. He balanced the three activity types in order to avoid a major pain flare in his arms. First, he alternated five minutes of dish washing (Pain Stressing Activity) with five minutes of reading (Pain Neutral Activity). After he did a couple of rounds of this, he decided it was time to increase his Comfort, so he sat in an easy chair and watched 30 minutes of a DVD with his arms wrapped in warm towels (Pain Relieving Activity). He eventually finished the dishes with minimal discomfort.

EXAMPLE BOX –
Margie's "Do Lists"

One Sunday, Margie decided to use the "Pay As You Go" Skill to pace her activities. She decided to plan her week by making a "Do List." First, she brainstormed the following set of tasks to carry out:

- ✓ Do two-loads of laundry
- ✓ Shop for food
- ✓ Get hair done
- ✓ Clean the bathroom
- ✓ Put some old photos in the new picture album
- ✓ Take car in for a tune-up
- ✓ Call her doctor about a question
- ✓ Meditate 20 minutes a day
- ✓ Exercise three times this week (walking in the park)
- ✓ Cook dinner three nights (husband & daughter cook other nights)
- ✓ Go to Comfort Skills Workshop on Wednesday

Next, Margie went through this collection and chose several high priority tasks to put on her **"A-List."** She prioritized them and it looked like this:

- ✓ Do two-loads of laundry
- ✓ Shop for food
- ✓ Go to Comfort Skills Class on Wednesday
- ✓ Meditate 20 minutes a day
- ✓ Exercise three times this week (walking in the park)
- ✓ Cook dinner three nights this week (husband and daughter cook other nights)

She put the rest of the tasks on a **"B-List."** These were important to do, but she didn't need to complete them as soon as the "A-List." The tasks included:

- ✓ Clean the bathroom
- ✓ Take car in for a tune-up
- ✓ Call her doctor about a question
- ✓ Get hair done
- ✓ Put some old photos in the new picture album

On Monday, Margie began to accomplish items on the "A List." She noticed that she got tired and achy mid-way through Monday. At that point, Margie decided to call it a day and rest. She appreciated the fact that she accomplished the following:

- ✓ Two-loads of laundry
- ✓ Shop for food
- ✓ Meditate 20 minutes a day

She'd also reminded herself that she would continue working on other "A-List" tasks on Tuesday. She noticed that by stopping when she did, she avoided the pain flares she used to get when she would Over-Do her tasks in the past. Margie had a pretty good night.

(B)
"The Payment Plan"

What happens if you want to do the "whole enchilada" with an activity? For example, you might desire to mow your entire lawn, clean the whole house, or go out and run around all day? Many of my colleagues would caution you against Over-Doing by suggesting that you should always pace yourself. However, what if you want to push your body beyond its comfort zone in order to perform a certain activity? In other words, what if you want to do something, from time to time, as if you had your Old Body? I differ from some pain specialists who tell you never to over-exert yourself. I believe that ***you can Over-Do on occasion as long as you plan to have a flare-up afterwards***. However, this is only for those of you who are willing to to push yourselves towards a pain flare.

MOVING SKILL BOX #3 –
"The Payment Plan"

Three Steps. For those of you who want to Over-Do an activity, use the following three steps to help you ride it out as comfortably as possible.

Step One – Plan to Have a Flare-Up. Acknowledge that if you Over-Do this activity, you'll probably get a pain flare. By admitting this, you have an opportunity to make one of two decisions:
   i.   Decide that it's not worth the extra pain and you'll drop it, or
   ii. Decide to Over-Do, and use the next two steps to ride out the flare.

Step Two – Delegate and Take Recovery Time. One way that an average pain flare turns into the "Mother of All Flares" is if you continue to Over-Do your activities after the pain flare starts. To avoid this, plan to take "Recovery Time" when the flare comes by resting your body, especially those parts most affected by the flare. Take time to soothe your body with well-earned down-time. Delegate your tasks to others who'll do them for you until you've fully recovered (or just put your tasks off 'til later). So, before you start to Over-Do, plan ahead and decide how you'll temporarily let go of your usual tasks (i.e., house chores).

Step Three – Use Your Skills. While you're laid up, you can distract yourself from the pain with a number of Enjoying Skills, such as naps, gentle stretching, music, movies, phone conversations, eating yummy (healthy) food, searching the Web, or by using Re-Focusing Skills such as Meditation or Hypnosis. Instead of drowning in waves of pain, use pleasurable distractions to surf over them.

STORY BOX #18 –
Cindy Rides It Out

For several years, Cindy suffered from low-back pain and migraine headaches. These limited much of her previously busy social life. However, her husband and three sons were planning a trip to a local amusement park and she was determined to join them. She decided to use the Payment Plan Skill to allow her to walk around the park for three hours. Cindy knew that she would have a two-day flare-up from this activity, but she planned to do it anyways *(Step One)*. Next, she told her family that she'd need their help and they offered it freely. She delegated her house responsibilities to her husband and kids so that she had time to recover *(Step Two)*. She also warned them that she might have to return from the park at a moment's notice if she felt a serious flare coming on. Her husband said that he'd give her a ride back and her teenage son volunteered to watch his siblings while his dad took Cindy home. She also called her boss and told him she had to take two sick days.

Cindy's recovery plan included lots of bed rest, meditation, movies, and special treats *(Step Three)*. She also had a new mystery novel and a list of people she wanted to call and write (Grandma wanted to know all the details of her Payment Plan). While she recovered at home, her family would stay at the park & later they'd all have dinner together (Dad would cook). The plan was set.

When the day came, she walked around the park for <u>four hours</u> and had a great time. Once she returned home, Cindy went to bed and used her distractions effectively to ride out the ensuing pain flare. Then, something curious happened – what would have been two days of flare turned into one! Cindy had a good time with her family, rode out the flare, and returned to a higher Comfort level faster than she expected.

Why Did the Pain in Cindy's Body Decrease so Quickly?

The answer is that she did three things that helped her to return to a comfortable equilibrium. First, she exercised the control that she had by planning for a possible flare-up. Pain wants you to think that you have absolutely no control over flares. However, Cindy and others have convinced me that there are many ways that you can gain some control of the situation. One is to choose when and where to have a flare up. As Cindy realized this, she was able to empower herself to plan for a flare and raise her Comfort to help her ride it out. This sense of control helped her to feel strong and prepared for difficulties.

A second reason that Cindy's pain flare faded was that she reduced her pain sensitivity by refusing to stress out or focus on the negative thoughts sent by Pain's cronies – Depression, Guilt, Anxiety, or Rage. For example, while she was watching a DVD, Guilt came along and put these condemning thoughts into her head: "What kind of mother are you?!" – You're just lying around like a lazy bum while the kids do your dishes!?" In her mind, she told him, "Go away! I'm too busy to think about you. I'm in the middle of a great movie." If she allowed her mood to drop, by listening to this Bad Guy, her pain sensitivity would have risen. Fortunately, she sent Guilt packing and desensitized her body by keeping up a positive mood.

Finally, Cindy gave herself time to rest and recover before and after she went to the amusement park. She combined this with a number of Comfort Skills (i.e., pleasure, laughter, meditation) that helped her to further calm her body, distract her from the pain, and successfully ride out the temporary discomfort. By exercising some control, increasing her positive mood, recovering with Comfort Skills, and resting before and after the outing, Cindy was able to shorten her time in the flare.

The Last Practice
"Breath Massage"
Use this Re-Focusing Skill for 20 minutes right now (see page 152).

HOMEWORK BOX
THIRD TRAINING DAY – WEEK 2

1. **Breath Massage.** During the days between now and the next week of training, practice the Breath Massage at least once each day. See if you can increase your practice by a few more minutes each time (see page 152).

2. **"Get Down & Laugh Me Thirty!"** Continue to use your own resources and the Laughter Boxes to laugh for 30 minutes a day (see pages 159 and 161).

3. **Imagine Spending Your Comfort Time.** Think about an activity you either Over-Do or Under-Do and consider how you might change it using one of the Moving Skills listed above. XTRA CREDIT – Apply one of the Moving Skills discussed above to an activity to either prevent Pain Flares or plan to ride it out.

4. **Notice Positive Change.** In the days between now and the next training week, notice large or small positive changes that enter your life by asking yourself:

    "What happened today, large or small,
    that I want to see more of in my life?"

Week Three – Sleeping, Meditation & Memory

Eight-Week Basic Training

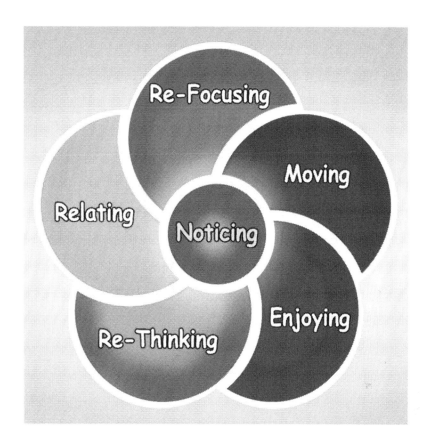

Pain Problems and Comfort Skill Solutions Included in Week Three

Pain Problems
- *"Poor Sleep and Rest at Night"*
- *"Attention Hijacked by Pain and Stress"*
- *"Sadness, Worry, & Other Miserable Feelings"*
- *"Hypersensitive Nervous System"*
- *"Poor Memory"*

Comfort Skill Solutions
- *"Day Skills for Night Sleep"*
- *"Rest in the Bed"*
- *"Work Back to Bed"*
- *"Mantra/Breath Meditation"*
- *"Look in the Book"*

WEEK THREE CONTENTS BOX

Sleep and Rest
First Training Day

1. The Skill Review
   A) *"Breath Massage"*
   B) *"I Want to See More of…"*
2. Today's Pain Problem
   ▪ *Pain Problem #3 – "Poor Sleep and Rest at Night"*
3. Learn/About #9 –Sleep, Rest and Chronic Pain
4. Skills of the Day
   A) *"Day Skills for Night Sleep"*
   B) *"Rest in the Bed"*
   C) *"Work Back to Bed"*
5. The Last Practice
   A) *"Breath Massage"*
6. Homework Box

Mantra/Breath Meditation and Stress
Second Training Day

1. The Skill Review
   A) *"Breath Massage"*
   B) *"I Want to See More of…"*
2. Today's Pain Problems
   ▪ *Pain Problem #2 – "Attention Hijacked by Pain and Stress"*
   ▪ *Pain Problem #9 – "Hypersensitive Nervous System"*
   ▪ *Pain Problem #4 – "Sadness, Worry, & Other Miserable Feelings"*
3. Learn/About #10 – Stress and Pain
4. Learn/About #11 - Meditation
5. Skill of the Day (and Last Practice)
   A) *"Mantra/Breath Meditation"*
6. Homework Box

Re-Thinking Memory
Third Training Day

1. The Skill Review
   A) *"Mantra/Breath Meditation"*
   B) *"I Want to See More of..."*
2. Today's Pain Problem
   ▪ *Pain Problem #12 – "Poor Memory"*
3. Learn/About #12 - The Re-Thinking Strategy
4. Learn/About #13 – How Memory Works
5. The Skill of the Day
   A) *"Look in the Book"*
6. The Last Practice
   A) *"Mantra/Breath Meditation"*
7. Homework Box

Sleep and Rest
First Training Day – Week 3

The Skill Review

(A)
"Breath Massage"

Practice this Re-Focusing Skill for 20 minutes (see page 152).

(B)
"I Want to See More of…"

Review your Journal or digital file, or recall the last couple days and answer these questions:

- **"What happened since the last Training Day, large or small, that I want to see more of in my life?"**
- **"What caused these things to happen?"**

Today's Pain Problems
Pain Problem #2 – "Attention Hijacked by Pain and Stress"
Pain Problem #3 – "Poor Sleep and Rest"

Learn/About #9 –Sleep, Rest, and Chronic Pain

Before Pain came along, most of you slept fairly well. However, a smooth running sleep pattern is disrupted by a combination of Pain, Depression, and Anxiety. A collection of scientific studies over the last two decades show that Pain and low moods will interfere with important sleep states and leave you exhausted in the morning[60]. What's worse, when you're deprived of sleep, pain flares increase in intensity and frequency[61] It's a kind of "Catch 22" in that poor sleep and pain increase each other[62].

Over the last century we have learned a great deal about sleep.[63] Sleep is significantly directed by a brain process called Circadian Rhythm. It greatly influences the quantity and quality of your sleep. The more stable and consistent your Circadian Rhythm functions, the better you sleep.

One way to understand the Circadian Rhythm is to imagine that you have a "clock in the middle of your brain." [64] Often, its setting enables you to ease into sleep at night and rise up refreshed and energetic in the morning with no problem. Over the years, many of you have not had any worries about resting at night because it happened naturally. In the past, some of you might have woken up in the morning before the alarm clock went off. However, on the weekend, many of you may have changed your sleep hours in order to stay up late at night and sleep late in the morning. When you did this, you threw off your internal clock – your Circadian Rhythm altered so much that it made getting up early for work on a Monday morning a very unpleasant experience!

So what happens to you if pain, depression, worry, multiple-medications, poor sleep habits, and other situations come into your life? The answer is that they "throw off your clock." Like memory, sleep is a very sensitive brain function that is altered by these

---

[60] Moldofsky, H (2001). Sleep and pain, Sleep Medicine Reviews, Volume 5(#5): Pages 385-96; Atkinson, J. H. and others (1988). Subjective Sleep Disturbance in Chronic Back Pain, The Clinical Journal of Pain, Volume 4(#4): Pages 201-270; Blau, J.N. (2002). Sleep Deprivation Headache, Cephalalgia: An international J of Headache, Volume 10(# 4): Pages 157-160. (Published Online).

[61] Lautenbacher, S, and others (2006). Sleep deprivation and pain perception, Sleep Medicine Review, Volume 10(#5): Pages 357-369.

[62] Roehrs, T, & Roth, T (2005). Sleep and pain: interaction of two vital functions, Seminars in Neurology, Volume 25(#1): Pages 106-116.

[63] See "The Promise of Sleep" by William C Dement, 2000.

[64] For more information, you can consult any text on sleep or do an online search for this term on Wikipedia or the Encyclopedia Britannica Online.

conditions. These problems can turn your nights into nightmares with only an exhausted morning to look forward to each day. Perhaps you experienced some or all of the following events during (and after) a bad night's sleep:

➤ Awake and aware of everything around you
➤ Tossing and turning in bed
➤ Eyes opened a lot
➤ Ears hear every little sound
➤ Breathing sometimes tight, sometimes fast
➤ Muscles are tense and you feel on edge
➤ Thinking is in high gear and often turns to worry and a focus on problems and tasks you need to deal with in the future
➤ Heart beats too fast to rest
➤ Sleep lasts only one or two hours at a time and you make multiple trips in and out of bed
➤ Feeling tired, low, and irritable in the morning and for the rest of the day
➤ Negative feelings like pain, depression, anxiety, and irritability increase

Given all of the above information, the most important question for you becomes: "What can I do to re-set my internal clock and get more sleep and rest?" Answers to this question will be presented in the sections below. It's divided into three sets of Sleeps Skills covering daytime and nighttime strategies.

Skills of the Day

(A)
"Day Skills for Night Sleep"

There are several Skills you can use during the day that will influence your night time sleep. Five of them are described in the next Box.

MOVING SKILL BOX #4 -
"Day Skills for Night Sleep"

1. **Avoid Stimulants Later in the Day.** Caffeine or Nicotine contain stimulating chemicals that can keep you up at night if you use them too close to bedtime. You can reduce their effect by stopping their use about six hours before bedtime (i.e., Stop drinking coffee at 3PM to go to bed at 9PM).

2. **Avoid Watching Intense Shows and Movies at Night.** Other "stimulants" that disturb your sleep at night are what you watch on a screen (i.e., TV, computer, smart phone, iPad). These keep you up because
   A) The light from your screen fools your brain into thinking that its "daytime" and that you should be awake (even after the show ends).
   B) The intensity of violent action or horror films, emotional dramas, thrillers, and the News will stress your body and make it difficult for you to get to sleep.

3. **Avoid Late or Long Daytime Naps**. A **Long Nap** is one that lasts longer than 30 minutes. A **Late Nap** can start sometime after 4PM. If you take a Long or Late Nap, there is a good chance that this will interfere with your night-time sleep (throwing off the accuracy of your internal clock).

4. **Light Control and Sleep.** Melatonin is a kind of "sleep hormone" produced in the Pineal gland located in the center of your brain. The Pineal Gland becomes active at night when things are dark. Scientists have found that you can use it to help you sleep at night by doing some of the following:
   A) *Face Sunning.* Get up early in the morning (between 6 and 8:30 AM) go outside and turn your face to the sun, or daylight, for 20 to 30 minutes. Protect your eyes by keeping them closed. Doing this may stimulate your Pineal Gland to excrete more of the sleep hormone Melatonin later on in the evening.
   B) *Increase Daytime Light.* Throughout the day, increase light by not wearing sunglasses unnecessarily, spending time outside during the daylight hours (i.e., eating lunch, exercising), increasing light in your home and workplace.
   C) *Decrease Night-Time Light.* Dim your house lights several hours before you go to bed.

5. **Setting Your Sleep Schedule.** This is one of the most powerful ways to improve your sleep. Simply decide when you want to regularly go to sleep at night and get up in the morning (i.e., 8AM wake-time and 11PM bedtime). These steps may help you do this:

- *Step One – Prepare Yourself.* Be ready for these temporary challenges:
  - ➢ A lack of sleepiness at the new bedtime.
  - ➢ Antsy feelings and tossing and turning in bed.
  - ➢ Feeling groggy after the alarm goes off in the morning. (Note - You'll need an alarm clock until you adjust.)

- *Step Two – Take Action.* Expect and do several things:
  - ➢ When these temporary challenges happen, prevent frustration by reminding yourself that "these will pass in time and I will be resting more easily in the near future."
  - ➢ Recall that if you feel sleepy during the day, you're likely to eventually fall into a deep sleep at your new bedtime.
  - ➢ Finally, if you find that it's hard to get sleep or rest at night, use the "Rest in Bed" or "Work Back to Bed" Skills (see below).

(B)
"Rest in the Bed"

This Skill is one way to calm the restlessness you feel in bed at night. It's based on studies that compared meditators and sleepers. In one experiment, researchers observed two groups of people, one that slept for eight hours and the other that meditated for two 20-minute sessions each day. The scientists looked at the brain waves each group emitted and found that the meditators' brains entered a sleep state similar to that of the eight-hour sleepers. Even better, the meditative brains registered the same amount of time in "Delta," which is a slow brain-wave associated with a good night's sleep. [65]

This is great news! If you can't sleep you have another option: You can rest by practicing any Re-Focusing Skill in bed ALL NIGHT LONG. Many of my workshop

---

[65] See the 1977 article in the journal, Psychophysiology entitled "Physiological changes in Yoga meditation," by B.D. Elson and colleagues, Volume 14, number 1, pages 55-57; the 1976 article in Science, "Sleep during Transcendental Meditation, " by R.R. Pagano and L.R. Frumkin, Volume 191, pages 308-309; the 1975 article in Perceptual and Motor Skills, Sleep during Transcendental Meditation, " by J. Younger and colleagues, Volume 40, number 3, pages 953-954.

attendees used one or more Skills, drawing from Breathing techniques, Imagery, Meditation, and Self-Hypnosis (all found in the Basic Training Program, Chapter Eight). When they did this, they either 1) fell asleep, or 2) comfortably rested throughout the night. In the morning, they all felt more rested and energized. The next Skill Box describes how you can do this.

MOVING SKILL BOX #5 -
"Rest in the Bed"

Step One – Give Up Sleep and Take a Rest. After 20 minutes awake in bed, give up sleep. Do not try to go to sleep that night; just rest.

Step Two – Turn Clock Around. If you are in the habit of looking at your bedside clock at night, you may have noticed that doing that will add to your stress and keep you awake. Free yourself from this by turning the clock around so you can't see its face.

Step Three – Rest in the Bed. Allow yourself to rest all night long by practicing the "Breath Count" and/or other Re-Focusing Skills (see pages 53 and 54 for a list of these Skills). If you fall asleep and wake up later in the night, repeat these Steps if you can't get back to sleep in twenty minutes.

Remember

- *"Replace Desperate Trying with Calm Noticing."* Be careful to avoid trying to go to sleep. "Trying" rarely works because most of us try too hard – and when we do we end up anxiously looking for a change. If good results don't happen immediately, we get upset, discouraged, and give up - or we try harder and become even more frustrated. Instead:
  - ➢ "Just do it to do it," and
  - ➢ Curiously notice what happens, instead of desperately trying to make things happen. Allow good results to come in their own time.

- *Adjust Yourself.* Feel free to adjust your body for Comfort as much as you want throughout the night, then refocus on the Skill practice.

(C)
"Work Back to Bed"

This Skill directs you to get out of your "tossing/turning bed" and do some work that'll eventually return you to a "sleepy bed." Although this may sound a little unusual it's very potent and differs from anything you've tried so far. It's based on the observation that the discomfort, irritation, stress, worry, and tension that you experience in bed generates a great deal of **Nervous Energy** that keeps you awake and on edge. The next Moving Skill Box will show you how to drain away that unwanted energy.

MOVING SKILL BOX #6 -
"Work Back to Bed"

Step One – Choose Your "Work." Pick a task to do at night that:
A) Will not irritate your pain condition
B) You can do over and over again, and
C) Is something you absolutely HATE to do

Step Two – Do it When You Can't Sleep. At night, if you're not asleep in 15 to 20 minutes, get up and carry out the activity you chose in Step One. Do it over and over until you get sleepy, then go back to bed.

Step Three – Back in Bed. Once you're in bed, you're likely to fall asleep. If you're still awake after 20 minutes, get up and do Step Two again until you're sleepy enough to return to bed. Repeat this step until you fall asleep.

How Does this Skill Help?

After reading that last Skill Box, you might think to yourself, "What is he talking about?! I'm annoyed enough by pain, low mood, and exhaustion, why put myself through this!?" The answer has to do with the Nervous Energy that's keeping you awake. Have you ever noticed that when you do your least favorite chore, you get tired, bored, and feel like you have to drag yourself through it until it's completed? This happens because when you engage in tasks that you hate to do, they deplete your energy. The good news is that you can use this on sleepless nights. When you can't sleep, you can use boring tasks to drain out the Nervous Energy that's keeping you awake and on edge. The following stories illustrate how this Skill works.

STORY BOX #19 - Charlie's Dishes

Charlie hated to do the dishes. When he decided to try the "Work Back to Bed" Skill, he left in the sink all of his dirty dishes. Predictably, when Charlie went to bed that night, he was still awake after 20 minutes. So, he got up, dragged himself to the kitchen, and began to clean the dishes. After he washed, dried, and put them away, he still felt awake, so he took the dishes off the shelf, put them back in the sink, poured vegetable oil all over them and washed them again! He did this several times before he felt tired enough to go back to bed. When Charlie returned to his bedroom, he collapsed into the bed and was surprised to find out in the morning that he slept several hours more than on other nights.

STORY BOX #20 - John's Fake Bills

John, an ex-contractor with a very painful back condition, tried this method to get more rest. He couldn't sleep more than an hour or two and had a hard time getting to sleep. One night, he got out of bed after 20 minutes of tossing and turning and did what he most hated to do - the bills. He hated to read them, make out checks, and put them in envelopes. Later, he even created a set of fake bills and checks and used them at night to "do the bills." It didn't take long before, exhausted, he fell asleep.

Last Practice
"Breath Massage"

Practice this Re-Focusing Skill for 20 minutes (see page 152).

HOMEWORK BOX
FIRST TRAINING DAY - WEEK 3

1. **Breath Massage.** Before the next Training Day, practice Breath Massage at least once each day. You will also benefit from practicing a little just before you go to bed (see page 152).

2. **"One Fun a Day!"** Do at least one thing each day that you enjoy.

3. **Practice "Rest In The Bed" or "Work Back to Bed."** Use the Sleep Skills above to increase your night-time rest and sleep.

4. **Spending the Comfort Time in Your Body Bank.** Apply the Moving Skills of "Pay-as-You-Go" or "The Payment Plan" to an activity that usually results in a pain flare (see pages 171 & 176).

5. **Notice Positive Change.** In the days between now and the next Training Day, notice any large or small positive changes that enter your life and write them down. Ask yourself each day:

> **"What happened today, large or small,**
> **that I want to see more of in my life?"**

Meditation and Stress
Second Training Day – Week 3

The Skill Review

(A)
"Breath Massage"
Practice this Re-Focusing Skill for 20 minutes (see page 152).

(B)
"I Want to See More of…"
Review your Journal or digital file, or think about the last several days, then answer these questions:

- **"What happened since the last Training Day, large or small, that I want to see more of in my life?"**
- **"What caused these things to happen?"**

Today's Pain Problems
Pain Problem #2 – "Attention Hijacked by Pain and Stress"
Pain Problem #9 – "Hypersensitive Nervous System"
Pain Problem #4 – "Sadness, Worry, & Other Miserable Feelings"

Learn/About #10 – Stress and Pain

Science has shown a clear relationship between the amount of stress you experience and the level of pain you feel. For some time now, health researchers have known about the debilitating and destructive effects of chronic stress.[66] Before learning the positive effects of Meditation, let's learn a little about how stress works. First, a couple of useful definitions:

A) **A Stressor** *is something or someone that challenges, frightens, and/or pressures you*

B) **Stress** *or the* **Stress Response** *occurs when we respond to that "something or someone" with fear, anger and other negative emotions.* **Usually it brings on the fight, flight or freeze reactions.**

When you feel threatened, you'll tend to jump into a "fight-or-flight" mode of action during which you'll prepare to either battle with the threat or run away from it. This causes

---

[66] http://www.mayoclinic.com/health/stress/SR00001

your nervous system to become extremely aroused and you'll either feel very angry and ready to fight or an overwhelming fear will either cause you to flee or freeze. You'll also experience an increase in your heartbeat, respiration, and blood pressure, and your muscles will tense up (see Table Box #1 below for a list of other stress-related effects). Many researchers believe that the current epidemic of High Blood Pressure, Heart Disease, and other stress-based illnesses are due to high levels of stress.[67] Unfortunately, stress also pumps up your sensitivity to chronic pain.

The Gazelle and the Lion

One way to illustrate the effects of stress is to imagine a typical scene from a nature documentary that shows a gazelle quietly eating grass in the savannas of Africa. Suddenly, a lion jumps out of the bush and hungrily runs to towards her. To save herself, the gazelle runs off and, as she does, her body starts to go through many changes designed to help her get away from the lion's devouring teeth. The following changes in the gazelle's running body are all good and necessary for such a situation:

- Stress hormones such as Cortisol and Epinephrine will pump into her body, releasing sugars that give her the energy to run fast, hard and long.
- Her heart rate and blood pressure increase to provide energy to her muscles.
- She tenses her muscles to move her body faster and faster.
- Her body redirects energy from her digestive system because she doesn't need to digest her lunch when she might become the lion's lunch.
- Her immunity shuts down because she needs the energy to avoid a lion, not a cold
- Her anxiety increases and that arouses her senses to look out for dangers as well as see and quickly run to escape routes.

If the gazelle escapes from the lion, she'll collapse, rest, and return to her normal physical condition. In such a case, stress would be very helpful for a mortally threatened animal.

The Stress Response is more complicated in humans. Although some stress is necessary to live, if it lasts too long, or is too overwhelming, it can "stress you out." One reason you stress out is because you have a large brain that has a powerful tendency to think about and imagine things. This process becomes an internal source of painful stress. If, for example, you took thirty minutes right now and imagined that you were being chased by a lion or some other threat, your body may respond like the gazelle in our example. Old memories can also set off a stress episode. So, if you focused on remembering your last major pain flare, you'd probably begin to feel uneasy and tense. In addition to your imagination and memory, internally focusing your attention on the pain itself can set off this kind of response.

---

[67] See "Why Don't Zebras Get Ulcers," by Robert Sapolsky.

You also may have external Stressors that set off this reaction. These include irritating friends or family members, annoying supervisors, co-workers, or other difficult people. For instance, one of my clients would predictably get a serious headache every time she took office work home with her. After about an hour of laboring at home (where she really wanted to rest), her head would start to throb and she's have to take a couple of days off work because of a searing migraine.

"Stress Hormone Soup"

If you feel overly stressed and remain sedentary day in and day out, you may experience a stress-related pain flare. As mentioned above, let's say you focused on a pain flare memory. If you fully immersed yourself in that memory, before long, some of those all-too-familiar pain miseries would return. And – if you stayed with that painful memory even longer, your body would fill up with Cortisol and other hormones and you'd become a living bowl of "stress hormone soup." What allowed the gazelle to return to a healthy normal physical state was that she burned off these hormones when she ran from the lion. Once she got away and rested, her body was clear of most of them. Unfortunately, many of you who are highly stressed tend to "freeze," that is you stay still and lie around, afraid to move, and while you're in bed or a chair, you'll fret over what worries you. That only increases your tension and fills you up with more stress soup.

The Pot, the Faucet, and the Burner.

Two ways to prevent yourself from filling up with stress hormone soup include: (A) Prevent these hormones from pouring into you, or (B) Burn off and evaporate them.

To understand this, imagine a soup pot with a faucet above pouring liquid into it. Under the pot is a stove burner. On the one hand, you can reduce the liquid in the pot by turning up the burner; this will evaporate liquid with heat. Similarly, when you've already been stressed out and you're full of Cortisol and other soup hormones, you can "evaporate" them by exercising. On the other hand, you can also shut off the faucet and stop the liquid from pouring into you. When you practice Re-Focusing or Enjoying Skills, you can prevent Stressors from releasing tress hormones into your body. In this section, you'll learn one way to shut the "stress faucet." It's a Re-Focusing Skill called Meditation.

TABLE BOX #1 **Harmful Effects from a Chronic Stress Response**	**TABLE BOX #2** **Beneficial Effects of Relaxation Response**

▪ Increased heart rate
 ▪ Hyperventilation
 ▪ Increases sugar levels in your blood (affecting Diabetes Two)
 ▪ Elevates blood pressure
 ▪ Lowers immunity to disease
 ▪ Increases pain sensitivity
 ▪ Raises muscle tension
 ▪ More depression & anxiety
 ▪ Irritability
 ▪ Increases bad habits and substance abuse (i.e., smoking)
 ▪ Increases over-eating
 ▪ Impairs memory
 ▪ Irritates skin conditions (ie, eczema)
 ▪ Stomach troubles
 ▪ Increase relationship conflict
	▪ Decreases heart rate
	 ▪ Calmer breathing
	 ▪ Returns to better sugar metabolism
	 ▪ Reduces blood pressure
	 ▪ Reduces muscle tension
	 ▪ Increases immunity and general health
	 ▪ Decreases pain sensitivity
	 ▪ Increases feelings of
	   ➢ Peace
	   ➢ Calm
	   ➢ Serenity
	   ➢ Contentment
	 ▪ Less depression and anxiety
	 ▪ Reduced bad habits and substance abuse
	 ▪ Greater alertness
	 ▪ Greater self-esteem
	 ▪ Improves relationships
	 ▪ Increases self-confidence

Learn/About #11 – Meditation

"Meditation" *includes "…a family of techniques which have in common a conscious attempt to focus attention in a non-analytical way and an attempt not to dwell on discursive, ruminating thought."*[68] Simply, Meditation is the practice of focusing your attention while noticing and letting go of distractions such as thoughts, feelings, and sounds. In this training program, Meditation is considered a Re-Focusing Skill. However, it originated from a variety of traditional spiritual and religious cultures from around the world. Over eighty years of research has found that this technique creates many positive physical and emotional benefits. On this Training Day, you will have the opportunity to learn one Meditation Skill.

We've come a long way since the 1950s when the average American knew very little or nothing about Meditation. Through the efforts of many scientists and healthcare providers, we have learned that Meditation is good for us because it has health benefits. Over the past thirty years, research has also revealed that the regular practice of meditation will help you to a) decrease pain, stress, and muscle tension, b) increase your quality of life, and, in some cases, c) reduce medication use.[69]

Two general types of Meditation you'll have a chance to learn in this training course are Single-Focus Meditation and one form of Mindfulness Meditation. Both are very useful. You can understand the difference between the two by imagining Meditation is like a camera lens.

Single-Focus Meditation – The Zoom Lens

Single-Focus Meditation *is the practice of settling your attention on a single (or combined) focus and doing your best to keep it there.* A few examples include a single focus such as the breath, a word or prayer quietly repeated in your mind, or the sound of a waterfall. Examples of a combined focus would be to direct your attention on your breath and on a word (i.e., "Calm") that you repeat quietly in your mind as the breath goes out. Some researchers call this "Concentrative Meditation" and they describe it as functioning like a zoom lens on a camera.[70] For example, let's say that you choose to focus on your breath. In Single-Focus Meditation, you'd "zoom in" on the feeling in your belly as you naturally inhale and exhale. While concentrating on the breath, you'd probably get distracted by thoughts, feeling, memories, or sounds. Each time this happens, you'd let go of the distraction and gently return your attention back to the breath. Later in this Training Day, you'll have the opportunity to learn one form of this practice called "Mantra/Breath Meditation."

---

[68] See "Meditation: Classic and Contemporary Perspectives," edited by Deane Shapiro, Jr & Roger Walsh.
[69] See "Full Catastrophe Living." By Jon Kabat-Zinn
[70] See 'The Physical and Psychological Effects of Meditation," by Michael Murphy and Steve Donovan.

Open-Focus Meditation – The Wide-Angle Lens

"Mindfulness Meditation" *is the practice of noticing and accepting, moment-by-moment, your thoughts, feelings, and sensations from the body and the surrounding environment while letting go of your tendency to judge or think about them*. Originally known as *Vipassana* Meditation, its believed to have developed 2500 years ago in Southern Asia.[71] It became popular in this country after the scientist and Meditation practitioner, Jon Kabat-Zinn, studied the effects of this practice on individuals just like you – people in chronic pain.[72] If Single-Focus Meditation works like a camera's zoom lens, Mindfulness Meditation functions like a "wide-angle lens." It's similar to Single-Focus Meditation in that you first "anchor" your attention to a single focus, such as a Mantra word or your breath. At the same time, you keep your awareness open to noticing whatever comes to mind. You'll notice thoughts, feelings, images, memories, sounds, and other mental distractions flowing through your consciousness. Often, they'll pull you away from your single focus. At this point, you become mindful of them and apply a number of techniques to keep your awareness either on the anchor focus or, like a wide-angle lens, on the whole scene in front of you.

Back to Single-Focus Meditation

In the next Box we'll learn a little about one of the early investigators and promoters of Single-Focus Meditation: Dr Herbert Benson, a founder and medical researcher at Harvard's Benson-Henry Institute for Mind Body Medicine.

INFO BOX #18 –
Dr. Benson's Relaxation Discovery

In the 1970's, Dr. Herbert Benson was particularly interested in studying a form of Meditation used by a new movement that had become very popular in many parts of the world: Transcendental Meditation. This was formulated by a spiritual teacher from India named of Maharishi Mahesh Yogi. It was based on an ancient practice called Mantra Meditation. Those who practiced this were instructed to repeat a "Mantra" (a special word) quietly over and over in their mind. Maharishi taught that you had to use the "correct" word, one that fit your spiritual energy. It was usually a sacred word from the ancient Indian language of Sanskrit. People who went through his training received such a Mantra and were told to "keep it secret."

---

[71] See "the Meditative Mind," by Daniel Goleman, and "Altered Traits: Science Reveals How Meditation Changes Your Mind, Brain, and Body," by Daniel Goleman and Richard Davidson
[72] See "Full Catastrophe Living." By Jon Kabat Zinn

This Guru was able to convince the public of the benefits of Meditation practice because he knew that most Americans believed in science. If a scientist discovers something good for us, we want it. So Maharishi hired reputable scientists to study his meditators and they found that Meditation reduced stress and increased a person's health and well-being. As a result of this and other factors, the popularity of Maharishi's meditation exploded and he attracted movie stars, business, and political people, and, for a while, the Beatles.

Dr. Benson was also interested in these health findings and he had a question: Did a person have to meditate on a special, secret Sanskrit word in order to benefit from meditation? He answered this by teaching college students to meditate on the word "one" and measuring the health effects. What did he find? – you guessed it! Benson found that when people meditated on any word (or any neutral or pleasant focus), their body would enter a different physical state that he called the "Relaxation Response" (see Table Box #2, above).

He made it possible for of people to practice a "secular" form of Meditation, one that also reduced chronic stress and its damaging effects (see Table Box #1). Interested individuals could enjoy the peace and serenity of this practice without having to attend a $300 seminar to learn a "secret word." Anybody could do it with any word.

The Relaxation Response

Recall the discussion we had at the beginning of this Training Day about the Stress Response. Dr. Benson's research findings suggest that Meditation prevents or pulls you out of a Stress Response. It can "shut the faucet" that usually releases stress hormones into your body. He and others have demonstrated that the effects of Meditation are essentially the opposite of those generated by the Stress Response.[73] He calls this the Relaxation Response and it provides many benefits (see Table Box #2, above). Other researchers have also identified many positive outcomes that derive from regular Meditation practice.[74]

Skill of the Day (and Last Practice)

---

[73] See http://www.psychosomaticmedicine.org/content/65/4/564.full
[74] See 'The Physical and Psychological Effects of Meditation," by Michael Murphy and Steve Donovan.

(A)
"Mantra/Breath Meditation"

Despite the fact that pain has dominated various parts of your brain, you can use Meditation to take them back. For example, when you focus on a physical sensation, such as the feeling of your breath moving in and out of the belly, you'll influence your brain's **Somatosensory Cortex**, the "Feeling" brain structure. When you focus your attention on the breath, it's as if you're temporarily moving pain signals out of that part of your brain.

Another meditative practice directs you to focus on a word that you repeat quietly in your mind over and over. This is called "Mantra Meditation" and when you practice it you'll influence your "thinking brain" structures called the **Pre-Frontal Cortex**. This is the area of the brain that is involved in thinking and is located just behind your forehead. When you repeat a Mantra (word) in your mind, over and over, you may experience fewer thoughts of worry, depression, or discomfort. If you meditate on both a Mantra <u>and</u> the breath, you'll focus two very important parts of your brain towards calm and Comfort. I call this method *"Mantra/Breath Meditation."* Like the "Breath Count" Skill, it builds up your Physical and Mental Concentration muscles.

RE-FOCUSING SKILL BOX #3
"Mantra/Breath Meditation"

Step One - Quiet Place and Timer. Find a quiet place to sit and set a timer for five or more minutes. Choose a seat or recliner that will comfortably support your body. Recall, if you lie down, you might fall asleep.

Step Two - Choose a Mantra Word. Choose a word or phrase that is positive, inspirational or calming. Examples -
   ▪ *Divine Names* - "Ribono Shel Olam," "Jesus," "Lono," "Allah"
   ▪ *Soothing Words* - "Calm," "Easy," "Serene," "Soothing," "Peace"
   ▪ *Hopeful Phrase* - "This Will Pass," "Feeling Fine," "Flowing Comfort"

Step Three - Practice the Meditation. Focus on the pairing of your natural breath with your chosen Mantra word or phrase. Each time you feel the breath go out, repeat the Mantra in your mind. If you wish, you can also repeat it when you inhale. Be sure to focus as much of your attention as you can on this practice.

Step Four – Let Go Into the Feeling. Many who practice this end up feeling pretty good. That feeling is like a bath of Comfort filling and surrounding you. When that happens, you can stop using the Mantra and redirect your attention onto the feeling alone - let it take you on a comfortable trip inside. Later, if you get distracted again by thoughts, uncomfortable feelings, or sounds, you can re-start your Mantra/Breath Meditation.

Step Five - Finishing. You can stop when your timer goes off. If you feel too good to stop, continue as long as you'd like until you're ready to return to the room by opening your eyes. Give yourself time to fully rouse yourself since you may feel very calm and relaxed. Walk around a little.

Bonus Meditation Option

As you focus on your in-breath, think the word, *"Deeply,"* and as you breathe out, think one of these words: *"Calm," or "Relaxed," or "Peaceful."* You might discover that this will allow you to focus even more closely and feel more at ease.

Remember

- **Let Distractions Be There and Re-Focus.** When a distracting thought, memory, image, feeling, sound, or anything tries to move your awareness away from the breath and the Mantra, just allow the distractions to stay there, like a quiet stream flowing by in the background. Don't fight them, simply "step out of the stream" and return your attention to the breath and the word.

- **Just Do It.** Free yourself from having to look for results or try to make something happen. "Just do it to do it" and notice what happens. Allow the comfort to come in its own time.

- **Adjust**. Feel free to adjust your body any time for comfort. If you find that you are moving around too much, take a break and practice later.

Okay, now sit for at least five to ten minutes and practice the "Mantra/Breath Meditation."

HOMEWORK BOX
SECOND TRAINING DAY - WEEK 3

1. **Mantra/Breath Meditation.** Between now and the next Training Day, practice this Skill at least once each day (see Box above for instructions).

2. **Have Fun Every Day.** Do at least one thing you enjoy every day. Use your "Fun Menu" (see page 163)

3. **Restorative Sleep and Rest.** Practice "Rest in Bed" or "Work Back to Bed" (on pages 186-188) to improve your night-time rest and sleep. *Xtra Credit* – If you would like to try on some of the "Day Skills for Night Sleep," go to page 185.

4. **Spend Your Comfort Time Wisely.** Apply the Moving Skills of "Pay-as-You-Go" and/or "The Payment Plan" to an activity that usually results in a pain flare (see pages 171-178).

5. **Notice Positive Change.** Between now and the next Basic Training Day, notice any large or small positive changes that enter your life and write them down. Ask yourself each day:

> "What happened today, large or small,
> that I want to see more of in my life?"

Re-Thinking and Memory
Third Training Day – Week 3

The Skill Review

(A)
"Mantra/Breath Meditation"
Practice this Re-Focusing Skill for 15 to 20 minutes (see page 198).

(B)
"I Want to See More of…"
Review your Journal, digital file, or think about the last few days and answer these questions:

- **"What happened since the last Training Day, large or small, that I want to see more of in my life?"**
- **"What caused these things to happen?"**

Today's Pain Problem
Pain Problem #12 – "Poor Memory"

Learn/About #12 – The Re-Thinking Strategy

"Re-Thinking Strategy" *is the practice of moving your thinking process away from forgetfulness and negativity and towards positive well-being.* It includes two forms: 1) Re-Thinking Memory, and 2) Re-Thinking Negative Thoughts.

As a wise man once said, "Whatever is on your mind, that's where you are." [75] The way you think has a profound effect on your mind and body. Problems of pain, illness, depression, and other difficulties get better or worse, depending on how you think about them. For example, if you take a hopeless view of pain, you might believe that your situation is an unending story of suffering, helplessness, and loss. Such beliefs and thoughts will increase your Misery level and often cause negative events to happen (i.e., a bout of depression or panic). By "Re-Thinking" and moving away from Negative Thoughts, you can make life better despite your painful challenges. By focusing on neutral or positive things in your life, you empower yourself to take control of your mind and brain. From there, you'll find opportunities to reduce your Misery and change some of the problems you face. In this Training Day, you'll learn about the first form.

---

[75] Rabbi Israel Ba'al Shem Tov, 18th Century.

STORY BOX #21 –
Bernie's Memory Problem

Bernie was only 43 years old but every time he forgot a doctor's appointment, he felt like he was ninety. His lapse in memory was caused by three of the "Big Eight Memory Blockers" (see next page).

These blocks were (1) **Physical Discomfort** brought on by a burning Neuropathic pain in his legs, (2) sedating **Side Effects** from the pain medications he took (i.e., Neurontin and Percocet), and (3) Poor concentration due to the **Low Mood** he felt.

All of these made it difficult for him to recall important things throughout his day.

In one session of the Comfort Skills Workshop, Bernie expressed his despair over his poor memory. Most of the group members bobbed their heads in agreement as he told story after story of how he couldn't remember to go to appointments, or to take his medication on time, or even to recall having met certain people. The incredibly sad thing about this is that Bernie used to work as a waiter in a high class restaurant and he prided himself on committing to memory every single order he received from customers. Ironically, one of the Big Eight Memory Blockers – Depression – would worsen when he thought about his forgetfulness.

Learn/About #13 – How Memory Works

As many of you probably know, ever since chronic pain came along, you've had a difficult time recalling information that used to be easy to bring up. Your ability to concentrate may also be less than it once was. This Learn/About will describe a little about how memory works, what blocks it and how to improve it.

The Big Eight Memory Blockers and How to Change Them.

As mentioned in the story above, there are eight major factors that interfere with your memory. The next two boxes will discuss these. Info Box #19 will present what I call the *"Big Eight Memory Blockers"* and briefly describe how each one interferes with memory. In Info Box #20 you will learn about a number of practices that counter each Blocker. Remember – you can locate the skills in "Appendix A," page 338.

INFO BOX #19 -
The Big Eight Memory Blockers

1) *Chronic Pain.* When the body hurts, it's difficult to focus on much of anything, especially on memory.

2) *Medication Side Effects.* You probably know that the sedating effects of many pain medicines will hamper your ability to concentrate and recall information.

3) *Low Moods.* When your mood moves into sadness, hopelessness, or outright depression, it becomes difficult for you to form or access memories.

4) *Stress and Anxiety.* When life stressors, such as money worries or annoying people, distract and upset you, it's hard to concentrate and remember.

5) *Disturbed Sleep and Rest.* It's been well established that your ability to remember is closely linked to the amount of sleep or rest you get in a night. Fatigue will increase forgetfulness.

6) *De-Conditioned Body and Mind.* Most people who suffer from chronic pain and emotional upset tend to reduce the amount of time they exercise their mind and body. When your mind isn't stimulated with reading, math, interesting documentaries, or other new learning, the brain is less able to recall things. Similarly, if you avoid physical exercise, your brain will receive less oxygen and this also inhibits your ability to remember.

7) *Social-Isolation.* One of the more interesting discoveries I've come across is how your social life affects memory. The less positive social connection you have, the more impaired your memory can become.

8) *Unhealthy Eating.* It's pretty clear that the average American diet (heavy fats and lots of processed sugars and other carbohydrates) is bad for your waist lines and cardiovascular systems. What you may not know is that it's also bad for your brain. Memory is also compromised by an unhealthy eating lifestyle.

INFO BOX #20 -
Changing the Big Eight Memory Blockers

1) Chronic Pain.

Goal: Increase your body comfort.

Skill: Surprise, surprise! – You can do this by practicing the Comfort Skills contained in this book!

2) Medication Side Effects.

Goal: Decrease sedating and other medication side effects.

Skill. Consult with your physician regarding a possible adjustment of your pain medicines and other prescriptions in order to reduce these effects. When you regularly practice Comfort Skills, you'll be better able to reduce some of your pills.

3) Low Moods.

Goal: Raise your mood to a happier place.

Skill: Use Re-Thinking Skills to change depressing thoughts. Re-Focusing and Enjoying Skills will also raise your mood and strengthen your positive thoughts and feelings.

4) Stress and Anxiety.

Goal: Building a sense of calm confidence and developing positive coping to reduce stressful situations.

Skill: Use Re-Thinking Skills to change Negative Thoughts that stress or worry you. Prevent these problems by using Moving Skills, especially those that reduce stressors in your daily life (i.e., pacing your activity level to reduce flares). You can also use Re-Focusing Skills like Meditation and Enjoying Skills like Laughter to bring calm in to your life.

5) Disturbed Sleep and Rest.

Goal: Increase sleep and rest at night.

Skill: Practice Sleep Skills.

6) De-Conditioned Body and Mind.

Goal: Strengthen body and mind.

Skills – Mind: There are numerous ways to exercise your mind. One rule of thumb is to study a variety of subjects and use different methods to learn them. These can include:

 ➢ *What?* A small list of general subjects that may include literature, math, science, art, religion, and philosophy. Pick things that interest you.

 ➢ *How?* Use different approaches to learning, including reading, watching science or history shows, searching the Internet, or attending classes and workshops.

 ➢ *Think Time*. Give yourself some time to think quietly, out loud, or on paper about any subject or idea you wish. Problem solving is another good thinking practice.

Skills – Body: For ideas on how to develop a physical exercise goal, join a gym, ride a bike, swim, or even take brief, regular walks. If you'd like, you can work with an exercise trainer or a physical therapist.

7) Social-Isolation.

Goal: Spend time with good people.

Skills: Redeveloping a positive, active social life.

8) Unhealthy Eating.

Goal: Learn how to eat more "brain health" food.

Skills: Consult a nutritionist, dietician, or Naturopathic doctor.

Skill of the Day

"Look in the Book"

Your ability to remember may improve when you create a source of memory outside of your brain. One analogy to explain this is the computer. Some of you who own a personal computer or laptop may have gone through the unfortunate tragedy of losing your data files because your hard drive "crashed." For those of you unfamiliar with "computer-speak," this means that the computer's memory library (the hard drive) breaks down and you are no longer able to access any of your documents, pictures, etc. One way to protect your files is to regularly save them on a memory source independent of the computer's hard drive. One form of this is called a "Flash-" or "Jump-" drive, which is a flat, plastic-covered device about the size of your pinky finger. When you plug it into your computer, you can copy your files onto it and, later, you can plug it into another computer and access your files.

What do you do if the brain, your "biological hard drive," is not working as well as before? One effective option is to put your most important information on an independent memory device – a "Memory Book." That's right, get yourself a blank journal or a weekly calendar, or create a special digital file on your smart phone, iPad, or computer and label it as your Memory Book. Write what you need to remember and later, when you want to recall something, <u>just look in the book</u> (or iPhone, etc.). That's it. This can be extremely helpful when you want to keep track of medications, tasks, appointments, and planned Skill practice times. The next Skill Box offers a few details as to how you organize and use your Memory Book.

RE-THINKING SKILL BOX #1 -
"Look in the Book"

Step One – Make a Memory Book. Purchase either a blank journal or a weekly calendar with plenty of room to write notes. Some of you may use a digital file on your smart phone, iPad, or computer.

Step Two - Organize and Fill Your Book. Decide what you want to include in the book and how you want to set it up. If it has a calendar format, record your appointments with their times under each date and use other blank space to list some of the following:

- A list of the things you want to accomplish that week.
- Important names and phone numbers.
- A collection of Comfort Skills that you want to practice.
- Other important ideas or tasks.

Step Three – Put it Where You'll See it. Before you go to bed, put your Memory Book in a familiar place in your house, one that you usually go to in the morning (i.e., kitchen table).

Step Four – Look in the Book. Begin your day at that familiar place in your home by looking through your Memory Book and recalling what you want to do that day. Example – One woman always left her Memory Book on her kitchen table at night. In the morning, while eating breakfast there, she'd look through the Book and review her day. Later, she'd put it in her purse and look at it, from time to time, throughout the day.

Option
- **The Back-Up Book.** Copy some of your important information into a second, "back-up book" or file in case you lose this one. Keep it in a familiar place.

The Last Practice
"Mantra/Breath Meditation"

For 15 to 20 minutes, practice this Re-Focusing Skill (see page 198).

HOMEWORK BOX
THIRD TRAINING DAY – WEEK 3

1. **Mantra/Breath Meditation.** Before you start the Fourth Training Week, practice this Focusing Skill at least once each day (see page 198).

2. **"Triple Fun."** Use your Fun Menu to do something you enjoy at least three times before the next Training Week (see page 163).

3. **Restorative Sleep and Rest.** Practice "Rest in Bed" or "Work Back to Bed" (on pages 186-188) to improve your night-time rest and sleep. *Xtra Credit* – If you would like to try on some of the "Day Skills for Night Sleep," go to page 185.

4. **Spend Your Comfort Time Wisely.** Apply the Moving Skills of "Pay-as-You-Go" and/or "The Payment Plan" to a different activity that usually results in a pain flare (see pages 171-178).

5. **Look in the Memory Book.** Use the Re-Thinking Skill Box above to improve your memory.

6. **Notice Positive Change.** In the days between now and the next Basic Training week, notice any large or small positive changes that enter your life and write them down. Ask yourself each day:

    "What happened today, large or small,

    that I want to see more of in my life?"

Week Four – Re-Thinking Negatives & Mindfulness
Eight-Week Basic Training

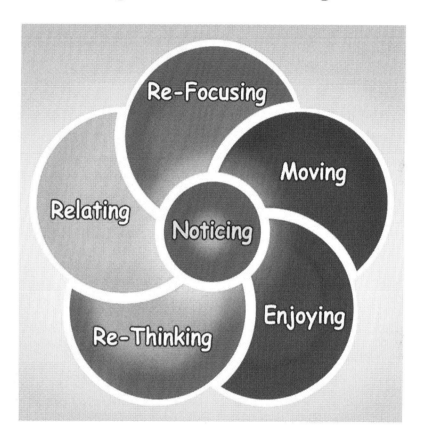

Pain Problems and Comfort Skill Solutions
Included in Week Four

Pain Problems
- *"Attention Hijacked by Pain and Stress"*
- *"Sadness, Worry, & Other Miserable Feelings"*
- *"Hypersensitive Nervous System"*
- *"Negative Thoughts"*

Comfort Skill Solutions
- *"Mindfulness/Thought Labeling Meditation"*
- *"See it Coming"*
- *"Remind Yourself About the Truth"*
- *"Talk Back and Step Aside"*
- *"Immerse in a Good Memory"*

WEEK FOUR CONTENTS BOX

Re-Thinking Negative Thoughts
First Training Day

1. The Skill Review
    A) *"Mantra/Breath Meditation"*
    B) *"I Want to See More of..."*
2. Today's Pain Problem
    - *Pain Problem #5 - Negative Thoughts*
3. Learn/About #14 – Re-Thinking Negative Thoughts
4. Skills of the Day
    A) *"See it Coming"*
    B) *"Remind Yourself About the Truth"*
    C) *"Talk Back and Step Aside"*
5. The Last Practice
    A) *"Mantra/Breath Meditation"*
6. Homework Box

Mindfulness Meditation
Second Training Day

1. The Skill Review
    A) *"Mantra/Breath Meditation"*
    B) *"I Want to See More of..."*
2. Today's Pain Problems
    - *Pain Problem #2 – Attention Hijacked by Pain and Stress*
    - *Pain Problem #9 – "Hypersensitive Nervous System"*
    - *Pain Problem #4 – "Sadness, Worry, and Other Miserable Feelings"*
3. Learn/About #15 - Mindfulness Meditation
4. Skill of the Day (and Last Practice)
    A) *"Mindfulness/Thought Labeling Meditation"*
5. Homework Box

Meditation Beads & Immerse in a Good Memory
Third Training Day

1. The Skill Review
    A) *"Laughing"*
    B) *"Mindfulness/Labeling Meditation"*
    C) *"I Want to See More of..."*
2. Today's Pain Problems
    ▪ *Pain Problem #2 – Attention is Hijacked by Pain and Stress*
    ▪ *Pain Problem #9 – "Hypersensitive Nervous System"*
    ▪ *Pain Problem #4 – "Sadness, Worry, and Other Miserable Feelings"*
3. Learn/About #16 - Meditation Beads
4. Skill of the Day (and Last Practice)
    A) *"Immerse in a Good Memory"*
5. Homework Box

Re-Thinking Negative Thoughts
First Training Day – Week 4

The Skill Review

(A)
"Mantra/Breath Meditation"

Practice this Re-Focusing Skill for 20 minutes (see page 198).

(B)
"I Want to See More of..."

Review your Journal or digital file, or think about the last several days and answer these questions:

> ▪ **"What happened since the last Training Day, large or small, that I want to see more of in my life?"**
> ▪ **"What caused these things to happen?"**

Today's Pain Problem
Pain Problem #5 – Negative Thoughts

Learn/About #14 – Re-Thinking Negative Thoughts

A **"Negative Thought"** *is any idea, belief, point of view, judgment, or mental image that increases your misery when you make it your focus of attention.* When you're dealing with Chronic Pain, you're likely to experience emotional discomfort. As I suggested in Chapter Two, you can imagine that this is brought on by "Bad Guys," such as Anxiety, Rage, and Depression, who send Negative Thoughts into your head. These create and worsen uncomfortable moods and body sensations. For example, Depression often likes to attack you with the harmful thought "I have no life." Unfortunately, if you believe this, you'll end up feeling quite low. Here is a Story Box that illustrates how Negative Thoughts may function in your life.[76]

STORY BOX #4 - Following Nothing

As a woman walked through town one day, she came across a stranger who held up a closed hand and said,

"In my hand is something that will change your life for the better. Do you want to see it?"

She said "yes" and followed him down the street, where he eventually came across a young man. The stranger held his fist up again and said,

"I have a wondrous thing in my hand that will positively change this woman's life and it can also change yours - would you like to see it?"

The young fellow agreed, and now the stranger had two people following him up one street and down another. After a while, he picked up ten more people with his promise. Eventually, he stopped walking and facing his little group he said,

"Okay, here is what you were all waiting to see."

He opened his hand and they saw...nothing. His hand was empty. The guy laughed and ran off. These people eventually realized that this trickster got them to follow him up one street and down another for nothing.

Following Negative Thoughts

---

[76] Story by Rabbi Nachman of Bratislav, see "Chassidic Masters and their Teachings," by Aryeh Kaplan.

Just like the trickster in the story above, destructive thoughts have no power over you unless you follow them. These toxic ideas work like con men on the street who try to manipulate you into seeing things their way. When you follow them, they lead to emotional places you don't want to go.

What can you do to prevent Negative Thoughts from making you miserable? You can "Re-Think" your situation. The Re-Thinking Skill described below will help you to ***"catch harmful thoughts before they catch you."*** Versions of this and other Re-thinking Skills were starting to develop over half a century ago by professional psychotherapists and researchers.[77] You can use the Skill to prevent yourself from following Negative Thoughts.

Skills of the Day
Three Re-Thinking Skills

Versions of the following three Rethinking Skills were developed over the last century.[78] Although you can use each one separately to catch and reduce Negative Thoughts, try using more than one to clear your mind and calm your emotions. The Summary Box below will briefly describe each Skill. This is followed by detailed Skill Boxes that show you how to "catch Negative Thoughts before they catch you."

SUMMARY BOX
THREE RE-THINKING SKILLS

Re-Thinking Skill One - "See It Coming." Since many Negative Thoughts tend to be repetitive, you can identify and notice them before they have a chance to annoy you.

Re-Thinking Skill Two – Re-Mind Yourself About the Truth. Negative Thoughts are lies or half-truths that upset you. When you recall what's true, you weaken these falsehoods.

Re-Thinking Skill Three - "Talk Back and Step Aside." Research has shown that when you quietly "Talk Back" to a Negative Thought in your mind, you reduce its impact. Also, when you "Step Aside," by distracting yourself with something positive, you'll stop Thoughts in their tracks, reducing Misery & pain.

---

[77] See "Handbook of Cognitive-Behavioral Therapies – Third Edition" by Keith S Dobson (Editor).
[78] Ibid.

(A)
"See It Coming"

As I've discussed earlier, Bad Guys like Depression and Pain influence you by sending negative messages into your head. If you follow these thoughts, they'll lead you into experiences that you probably want to avoid (i.e., depressed mood, increased pain awareness, over-eating, muscle tension). Cognitive-Behavioral psychologists and other practitioners have created a variety of Skills that help you notice and interrupt Negative Thoughts and harmful attitudes.

I call one of these **"See it Coming,"** and it helps you to catch destructive thoughts before they have a chance to seduce you into following them. As you notice their irritating patterns and harmful messages, you'll stop them in their tracks and prevent a lot of Misery.

STORY BOX #5 - The Snowball Demon

Jacob, a friend of mine, told me that he first learned how to "See it Coming" from his ten-year-old cousin Arnie, the "snowball demon." He'd visit Arnie in wintertime Colorado and, as usual, they'd get into a snowball fight, which ended with Arnie burying Jacob under an avalanche of ice. However, when Jake turned thirteen, he began to notice <u>how</u> Arnie threw his "snowball sandwiches."

Jacob noticed which direction the balls came from, where they hit, the faces Arnie would make before he threw one, how he stood, how big the balls were, etc. After a short while, and a lot of snowballs, he could predict where the balls would go and he easily avoided them. After that, Arnie ate all the snowball sandwiches!

Just as Jacob saw the snowballs coming, you can see Negative Thoughts coming, and take action to block them. When Depression sends his sad and hopeless messages into your head, he wants you to believe that they come from you. That's what makes the thoughts so believable. You can separate yourself from these hurtful ideas by reminding yourself that, for the most part, you didn't have a lot of Negative Thoughts before Pain and other Bad Guys entered your life (or at least not as many. The next Re-Thinking Info Box will be followed by this Skill Box.

INFO BOX #15 -
Common Negative Thoughts

- "I'm such a cripple."
- "This will never change."
- "My life is over."
- "It's going to get me no matter what I do!"
- "I'm such a burden on everyone."

RE-THINKING SKILL BOX #2 -
"See it Coming"

Step One - Notice Them. Over the next week or two, each time you notice that you're in a low mood or anxious state, observe what kind of Negative Thoughts were in your mind before you felt bad. For example, Thoughts such as "I'm such a disappointment to others" or "I can't do anything anymore." (If that's too difficult to do when you're feeling distressed, wait until your mood improves, then recall what thoughts came along before you felt so bad).

Step Two - See It Coming with a Friendly Warning Phrase. After you've identified the Negative Thought, notice it whenever it shows up and repeat in your mind a phrase such as
- "There he goes again!"
- "Not you again!"
- "Look who is back."
- "There's that _____ (i.e., depressing) thought from yesterday."
- "Haven't I seen you someplace before?"

Step Three - Set It Aside. After you notice the Negative Thought and say your Friendly Warning Phrase, mentally set the Thought aside and go about your daily business. If you have to repeat your Phrase several times before you can let the Thought go, that's fine.

This next story describes how one person in pain fended off the Negative Thoughts that her husband tried to put into her head.

STORY BOX #6 - Marcia Sees It Coming

I once counseled a woman named Marcia whose husband would often say terrible things to make her feel guilty. Usually, they had a good relationship, but her husband's periodic "guilt tripping" was very annoying. What's worse – she'd fall for it every time by feeling horrible and it left her feeling miserable and depressed. In a way, <u>she was allowing him to put his Negative Thoughts into her head</u>.

"He gets very obnoxious and repeats the same lines over and over and I listen to it," she told me with much frustration. Marcia admitted that she wanted to stop these words from affecting her. I suggested that once she saw his guilt words coming, she could say a funny word or sentence quietly in her mind, then ignore him. Soon after our session, her husband came home and told her, "You never get dinner to the table on time and you know how this throws off our family schedule!" She immediately "Saw it Coming," and recognized that this was the same old stuff he'd throw at her when he was tired and cranky from his day. She then said to herself, "<u>There he goes again!</u>" and laughed about this a little on the inside. When Marcia continued preparing dinner and ignored his tantrum, he quieted down.

Later she told me that this Skill worked like a charm and it prevented Guilt from bringing her down. What was even better - as she continued to meet her husband's guilt tripping with this Re-Thinking Skill, he did it less and less.

Although this example involved a real person, you can do the same with the Negative Thoughts that come into your mind. You can use See It Coming to disarm them. When you do this, you may experience two things:

- ❖ **First**, you'll feel more in control because you caught the thought before it caught you.
- ❖ **Second**, you might laugh at the thought and at the Bad Guy who sent it. As you giggle on the inside, perhaps you'll say things to yourself like "There he goes again, what an obnoxious Butt-head! Does Anxiety really think he can get away with <u>that</u> lie again!"

Overall, the more you "See It Coming," the easier it gets to catch a Negative Thought before it catches you.

(B)
"Re-Mind Yourself About the Truth"

Negative Thoughts act like some lawyers and politicians – they lie. Or, at best, they express half-truths that are worse than lies because they sound true. For example, one woman I worked with was troubled by the Negative Thought, "I'll never play golf again. I'll just be stuck at home in Misery while my golf partners have fun." This Thought depressed her. Fortunately, when she realized that it was possible to "Do It Differently," the woman arranged to join her friends (who were very supportive), play three out of the eighteen holes, then followed her girlfriends in a golf cart. By the end of the afternoon, they all got together for a great lunch and good conversation. Remember, just as this story shows, Negative Thoughts are lies, lies, lies! Use them to remind you that you can discover what is really true.

The opposite of a lie is the truth. You may be familiar with the teaching from Christianity, other religions and philosophies that "the truth will set you free." When it comes to freeing yourself from the grip of Negative Thoughts, this is quite true. There are several truths that apply to your situation. When you use the Skill Boxe below, it will guide you as to how to "Re-Mind Yourself About the Truth" when Depression, Anxiety and other Bad Guys flood your mind with lies.

INFO BOX #21 -
Common Truths about You and Pain

1. When you feel pain, it's not your fault.
2. As a person-in-pain, you have nothing to be ashamed of.
4. Most of you are not a drug addicts.
5. You can change your mind.
6. You can feel helpless and know that you are not helpless.
7. You don't have to follow a Negative Thought.
8. Flare-ups eventually flare-down and you'll return to a comfortable state.
9. There are things that you can do to increase your Comfort

RE-THINKING SKILL BOX #3 -
"Re-Mind Yourself about the Truth"

Step One - Identify the Lie. Notice what kind of Negative Thought is upsetting you. Example - Hopelessness sends you the thought, "Nothing will ever get better."

Step Two - Dig for the Truth. Recall events and personal qualities that contradict that lying Negative Thought. Example – One person noticed the thought "I have no life" was in her head. She took some time and remembered how she engaged in a number of life-affirming activities that week, including playing with her nephew, taking a pleasant walk with her sweetheart, and reading an interesting book. She also recognized that all of these activities were part of "having a life," a very powerful truth for her.

Step Three - Use a "Truth Journal." If you have a difficult time recalling the truths about yourself that counter the lying Negative Thoughts, you can get a blank Journal or digital file and designate it as your "Truth Journal." Record some of the Negative Thoughts that bother you and list the truths that counter them. It's useful to read this Journal from time to time.

STORY BOX #22 - "Fat" Betsy

Thirty-seven-year-old Betsy noticed that whenever she looked into a mirror, she'd hear the thoughts of Guilt accusing her of being "fat and lazy" (a very hurtful insult for an ex-model). After she identified this lie, she Dug for the Truth and reminded herself that she had recently begun an exercise program at the gym, which increased her activity level. Next, she acknowledged that she already lost a couple of pounds. She also remembered that having a disability, which limited her activity, did not mean that she was "lazy." In fact, she was pretty active for someone who, only a couple of years ago, fell backwards down 15 concrete steps. Finally, she recognized that the word "fat" was an insult she could ignore.

By reminding herself about these truths, she was able to reduce the lies she heard from Guilt and Depression, and that increased her mood and confidence so that she was able to take on more activities. Doing this helped Betsy to feel better about herself and to experience more Comfort in her day.

You Don't Have to Follow the Thoughts

Here are two basic truths you can Re-Mind yourself about: First, recall that **Following a Negative Thought causes a low mood or bad habit to follow you,** and second, you can avoid these Thoughts by Re-Minding yourself that when they enter your head, **you don't have to follow them.** Instead, give yourself permission to let them pass.

(C)
"Talk-Back and Step-Aside"

Talk-Back

One of the most potent weapons you can use against Negative Thoughts is to quietly "Talk Back" to them in your mind. Your forceful, positive counter-thoughts will cut down most negative messages over time.

Step-Aside

After you've talked back to the Negative Thoughts, give yourself some time to "Step Aside" by engaging in an activity that redirects your attention towards something neutral or pleasant, like walking, a movie, or a phone call. When you do this, it's as if the Thought is shooting towards you and you turn aside, causing it to pass you by.

In the next Skill Box, you'll learn how to do this. Betsy's second Story Box will illustrate how she used this Skill

---

RE-THINKING SKILL BOX #4 -
"Talk Back and Step Aside"

Step One – "Talk Back." Create a couple of "one liners" that can interrupt the Negative Thoughts that bother you. Say them in your head as many times as you need. Example - Talk-Back lines may include:
- "I'm not going there!"
- "Forget about it!"
- "No way!"
- "I don't need to listen to you."
- "I got through this before and I can do it again!"

Step Two – "Step Aside." After you Talk Back to the Negative Thought, use items listed on your "Fun Menu" to distract you from the Thought. Example – you may want to do one of the following:

- Take a pleasant walk
- Call a friend
- Watch a movie or read a book
- Hang out in the garden
- Play a game

"Talk Back and Step Aside" – An Example

When George felt a flare coming on, Panic would send him this Negative Thought, "I'm going to fall apart!" He immediately did the following:

- *Talk Back.* He countered Panic by thinking, "Oh no I'm not, I'll get through this!"
- *Step Aside.* He put himself in a comfortable position and listened to a relaxing CD. Later, he watched a movie as he sat in his easy chair and followed that with a brief walk.

STORY BOX #23 - Betsy Puts Them in the Middle

We met Betsy in the previous Story Box. She was a very successful, thirty-something, African-American model and assistant manager at a popular clothing store on the day she fell down a set of concrete steps, damaging her back and neck and turning her life into a living hell. Between constant pain and a debilitating depression, she lived under the shadow of Misery and doom.

When I first began to work with her, she was contemplating suicide. Several months later, she came into my office and surprised the heck out of me - she was smiling! When I commented on this she told me the following:

"Recently, I got tired of Depression and Pain telling me that I had no reason to live. I realized that all this time, they were putting me in the middle of a circle of Misery and were trying to suffocate me there. All that is changed now because I put Pain and Depression in the middle and I'm all over them! Here's what I do: When they send their evil thoughts into my head, I put up my hand like I'm pushing them away and I say in my mind: '<u>I'm not going there</u>! No way, not with you!' Then I leave them behind by doing something like watching my favorite soap opera or taking a little walk."

Although a version of what she discovered on her own was also developed by psychologists, it was even more satisfying for me to hear that she figured out on her own how to use keep depression out of her life.

When I last spoke with Betsy, she was lighting up her life through new activities, friends, and attending community college.

The Last Practice
"Mantra/Breath Meditation"

Practice this Re-Focusing Skill for 20 minutes (see page 198).

HOMEWORK BOX
FIRST TRAINING DAY – WEEK 4

1. **Mantra/Breath Meditation.** Before the next Training Day, practice this Focusing Skill at least once each day for 20 minutes (see page 198).

2. **"One Fun a Day!"** Do at least one enjoyable activity each day using your "Fun Menu" (see page 163).

3. **"See it Coming."** Use this Rethinking Skill Box to identify some of the most common Negative Thoughts that go through your mind. Write these in your journal (see pages 215-216).

4. **"Re-Mind Yourself About the Truth."** Choose a Negative Thought that often lies to you and recall a truth that counters it (see pages 218-219).

5. **"Talk Back and Step Aside."** Recall some of the most common Negative Thoughts that annoy you and plan to confront them by using this Re-Thinking Skill (see pages 220-221).

6. **Notice Positive Change.** In the days between now and the next Training Day, notice any large or small positive changes that enter your life and write them down. Ask yourself each day:

   **"What happened today, large or small,
   that I want to see more of in my life?"**

Daniel Lev

Mindfulness Meditation
Second Training Day – Week 4

The Skill Review

(A)
"Mantra/Breath Meditation"
Practice this Focusing Skill for 20 minutes (see page 198).

(B)
"I Want to See More of…"
Consult your journal or digital file or think about the last several days and answer the two questions below.

- "What happened since the last Training Day, large or small, that I want to see more of in my life?"
- "What caused these things to happen?"

Today's Pain Problems
Pain Problem #2 – Attention Hijacked by Pain and Stress
Pain Problem #9 – "Hypersensitive Nervous System"
Pain Problem #4 – "Sadness, Worry, and Other Miserable Feelings"

Learn/About #15 – Mindfulness Meditation
As described in Learn/About #11, **"Mindfulness Meditation"** *is the practice of noticing and accepting, in each moment, your thoughts, feelings, bodily sensations, and the surrounding environment while you let go of your tendency to judge and think about them.* This Skill is a very ancient and scientifically well-established method to help people-in-pain reduce stress and raise their Comfort level in the face of Misery and discomfort. In the late 1970s, Dr. Jon Kabat-Zinn's research revealed the power of "Mindfulness Meditation" to modify the pain experience.(see his book, "Full Catastrophe Living"). This form of Meditation has recently been adopted by many medical centers as a standard training for people suffering from pain, depression, anxiety, and other stress-related difficulties. In the training below, you'll learn one form of this powerful technique.

In order to better understand how to practice this Skill, you'll first find it helpful to learn about "Distracting Thoughts" and "Thought Labeling."

Distracting Thoughts

Many things that disturb you are related to thoughts. For example, let's say that you hear a door slam in your apartment complex while you're home listening to music. After the initial slam, if you continue to feel bothered by the sound, it's not the noise that sidetracks you – it's your thinking about it (i.e., you might think over and over, "Can't those people be quiet!!").

The same thing happens with uncomfortable feelings. Once you notice them, you may become focused on thoughts that "talk" about them. These Negative Thoughts can bother you even more than the painful sensations that started them. For example, if you feel a shock of pain go through your back, you might notice thoughts flowing through your mind such as the following:

- "Damn, I hate when that happens."
- "There it goes again, what's it gonna do now?!"
- "When in the hell will this damn pain stop!"
- "G-d Dammit! Where's my Norco?"

Thought Labeling

This is one of a number of Mindfulness techniques that you will find useful. **"Thought Labeling"** *is the Mindfulness Meditation practice of noticing and mentally naming a distraction each time it comes along and then returning to focus.* Often, the word *"thought"* is used to name these distractions. Labeling is a very powerful way to reduce the negative influence of distracting thoughts. The goal is to help you catch them before they push you into miserable, pain-exacerbating rumination.

How does Thought Labeling help? Briefly, the goal of Meditation, and most of the Re-Focusing Skills, is <u>not</u> that you should stay focused all of the time. That is not possible because our brains will inevitably distract us with a thought, image, feeling, etc. Even some Buddhist Monks are limited: Although they have meditated for hours a day over many years, these dedicated practitioners (according to one study) can only stay focused for about thirty seconds before they get distracted.

It's all about memory. When we get distracted by one thought, it leads to many others that cause us to forget our practice goal to stay as focused as we can and relax our bodies. For example, if I'm meditating on my breath and the thought "what's for dinner?" comes into my head, I'm liable to forget what I'm doing and start considering other thoughts like, "I could take a steak out of the fridge," "I can cook up some potatoes and carrots," "Maybe I can invite someone over for dinner," and "Wow, that dinner I had at Cindy's house last weekend was great!" This is all fine, but I forgot that I'm trying to focus on my breath.

When I'm distracted like that, the real goal of Meditation (and other Re-Focusing Skills) <u>is to help me remember what I'm doing</u> by "re-focusing" my attention back to the breath (or some other focus). "Mindfulness/Thought Labeling Meditation" helps you do that by directing you to label the distractions that hijack your attention with the word "Thought." Since we're more distracted by our thoughts about a distraction, like noise, we label all distractions as thoughts.

Skill of the Day (and Last Practice)

FOCUSING SKILL BOX #4 -
"Mindfulness/Thought Labeling Meditation"

Step One - Quiet Place and Timer. Find a quiet place to sit and set your timer for twenty minutes. Choose a seat or recliner that will comfortably support your body.

Step Two - Choose and Meditate on a Focus. Select a focus that's pleasant or neutral, such as a Mantra word or your breath (for more, see the Info Box below). Concentrate your attention on this focus and keep it there as best you can.

Step Three - Thought Labeling. Eventually, a distracting thought, memory, sensation, image, feeling, or sound will come along and draw you away from your focus. When this happens, mentally label it with the word "thought" and then return your concentration back to the focus. Do this for every distraction, even if it is not an obvious thought (i.e., a door slamming).

Step Four - Finishing. Stop when your timer goes off. Take time to fully arouse yourself since you may feel very calm and relaxed. Walk around.

Remember
Don't look for results, "just do it to do it" and see what happens. Allow the comfort to come in its own time.

INFO BOX #22 -
Things to Concentrate on During Meditation

Visual Focus
- Candle flame
- Flower or plant
- Ocean waves, flowing stream
- Picture

External Sound Focus
- Recorded sound of rain, flowing water, soft music
- Natural sounds such as ocean waves
- Gentle instrumental music

Internal Sound Focus
- Mantra (word sounded in your mind)
- Quiet prayer
- Remembering a number of songs and replaying them in your mind

Physical Sensation
- Belly moving in and out as you breathe
- A comfortable part of your body
- An object or activity (rubbing a smooth stone, or taking a slow walk)

HOMEWORK BOX
SECOND TRAINING DAY – WEEK 4

1. **Mindfulness/Thought Labeling Meditation.** Over the next several days, practice there- Focusing Skill above at least once each day for 20 minutes.

2. **"One Fun a Day!"** Do at least one thing each day that you enjoy using your "Fun Menu" (see page 163)

3. **Notice Positive Change.** In the days between now and the next Training Day, notice any large or small positive changes that enter your life and write them down. Ask yourself each day:

   **"What happened today, large or small,
   that I want to see more of in my life?"**

Meditation Beads and

Immerse in a Good Memory
Third Training Day – Week 4

The Skill Review

(A)
"Laughing"

Take 30 minutes and practice "Laughing" by watching funny TV shows, movies, stand-up comedy, or wild three-year-olds dancing! (See page 159.)

(B)
"Mindfulness Meditation/Thought Labeling"

After laughing, practice this Skill for 20 minutes (see page 226).

(C)
"I Want to See More of…"

Consult your Journal, or review the last several days and answer these questions.
- **"What happened since the last Training Day, large or small, that I want to see more of in my life?"**
- **"What caused these things to happen?"**

Today's Pain Problems
Pain Problem #2 – Attention Hijacked by Pain and Stress
Pain Problem #9 – "Hypersensitive Nervous System"
Pain Problem #4 – "Sadness, Worry, and Other Miserable Feelings"

Learn/About #16 – Meditation Beads

There are a number of ancient cultures and spiritual traditions that advocate the use of a string of beads for meditation and prayer. The Buddhists, Hindus and Sikhs call them Japa Mala or Mala beads, and some Muslims refers to it as a "Tasbih." As is well known in the West, Catholics use the Rosary beads in their religious devotions. Whether spiritual or secular, all people can receive health benefits from the use of meditation beads. Two advantages of using beads as part of your meditation practice include time-keeping and brain stimulation.

The "Timer"

As you see in the picture below, each string of Mala beads has one large or distinct bead at one end. Practitioners usually start with the smaller bead that comes after this large bead. Each time they notice the breath going out and/or they repeat a Mantra word in their mind, they gently move a bead down with their thumb. When they've made one circuit and return to the large bead they'll have spent a certain amount of time meditating (the first time you do this, look at the clock before you start and after you reach the bog bead and you'll know how long one circuit takes). Thus, the Mala beads serve as a "timer" that allows you to fully concentrate on your Meditation without having to look at a clock. Once you know how long it takes to move around the entire set of beads once (i.e., five minutes), you can decide how many circuits you'd like to practice that day.

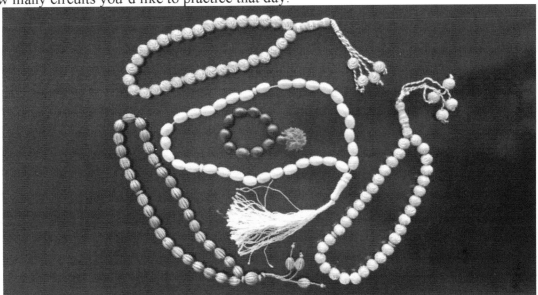

Mala (Meditation) Beads

Stimulating Your "Action Brain"

In addition to being a useful timing device, the Mala beads also benefit you in another way. First, let's review what happens in your brain when you do Mantra Meditation. Remember that a Mantra is a word or phrase that you repeat in your mind over and over. This redirects your attention towards one thought (the Mantra word) and away from uncomfortable ideas or feelings. When you do this, you're stimulating and focusing your "Thinking Brain," or Pre-Frontal Cortex located behind your forehead. Let's say that as you sound the Mantra in your mind each time you also focus on your breath exhaling. As you do that, you're also focusing on the feeling of the breath as it moves in and out of your belly. That engages the "Feeling Brain," or Somatosensory Cortex located in the middle-rear of the brain.

What happens in the brain if you simultaneously move a Mala bead whenever you repeat a Mantra while breathing out? The answer is that you stimulate the top-middle slice of the brain called the Motor Cortex, or the "Action Brain." All together, when you use the

229

Mala beads in this way, you'll focus three functions of your brain on the Meditation and this re-routes some of your energy and attention <u>away</u> from pain and emotional distress and towards peace and comfort. Because you can gain even more influence over three parts of your brain, I recommend that you enhance your Meditation sessions with meditation beads.

Skill of the Day (and Last Practice)

"Immerse in a Good Memory"

When you "Immerse in a Good Memory," you take time to replay some of your best memories in your mind and fully re-experience and enjoy them (Positive Psychologists call this "Savoring").[79] As you do this you may feel like you're immersing in a happy bath.

RE-FOCUSING SKILL BOX #10 - "Immerse in a Good Memory"

Option One - Immerse While It's Happening. When you're engaged in a pleasant, ecstatic, or fun activity, allow yourself to completely focus on all of its tastes, smells, sights, and sounds. When you get pulled away by thoughts or distractions, let them go, return to immersing in your pleasurable moment.

Option Two - Immerse in a "Fun Re-Run." What can you do if you're not engaged in something fun right now? Draw on your memory of past enjoyable activities (i.e., perhaps some written in your "Good Stuff Journal," see page 254). Just sit or lie comfortably, recall a great experience you've had in the past, and let yourself re-live it in your imagination. Allow yourself to re-experience all the tastes, smells, sights, and sounds of the activity that you recall. Two ways to do this are as follows:

- *Watch the Movie.* Re-live your happy experiences by imagining that you're at the movies watching it happen on the big screen. It's like you're re-playing inside your head a great movie from your life.
- *Enter the Movie.* Imagine yourself stepping into that big screen movie and re-living your story.

---

[79] See "Savoring: A New Model of Positive Experience," by Fred B. Bryant and Joseph Veroff, (2006).

STORY BOX #24- Alice Leaves Panic Behind

Alice was beginning to succumb to a Panic Attack one day after she sat in my office recliner. Immediately, I asked her if she would like to feel better and she said yes. I invited her to close her eyes, keep breathing deeply, and remember a safe, comfortable experience she had in the past. She did so and in less than 90 seconds, she opened her eyes calmly and said that she felt a lot better. When she immersed in the warm memory of her honeymoon in Hawaii, the Panic vanished.

Okay, now take fifteen minutes and practice "Option Two" in the Skill Box above.

WEEK FOUR
"HALF-TIME" HOMEWORK & SKILL REVIEW BOX
THIRD TRAINING DAY – WEEK 4

1. **Re-Focusing "Variety Pack."** During the days before you start Week Five, practice any of the Re-Focusing Skills you've learned so far. You might choose to use several or only stick with one:
   - *"Breath Count"* (see page 130)
   - *"Breath Massage"* (see page 152)
   - *"Mantra/Breath Meditation"* (see page 198)
   - *"Mindfulness/Thought Labeling Meditation"* (see page 226)
   - *"Immerse in a Good Memory"* (see page 230)

2. **"One Fun a Day."** Do something you enjoy at least once a day before the next training week. Use your "Fun Menu" (see page 163).

3. **"Laugh Right Now!!"** Take some time and use the Laughing Skill Boxes to giggle for about 30 minutes each day (see page 159).

4. **Re-Thinking Skills.** Continue these to deal with Negative Thoughts (see pages 215-221):
   - *"See It Coming"*
   - *"Re-Mind Yourself About the Truth"*
   - *"Talk Back and Step Aside"*

---

5. **Noticing Triggers and First Signs.** Use these Skills to identifying the Negatives that warn you about pain flares before they come on strong (see pages 148-149).
   - *"Revealing Triggers"*
   - *"Revealing First Signs"*

6. **Use Your Body Bank for Comfort.** In order to avoid or ride out pain flares, continue to use the following Skills found on pages 171-176.
   - *"Pay as You Go"*
   - *"The Payment Plan"*

7. **Create a New Future.** If you are plagued by Under-Doing, recall that ***"Setting a Goal"*** will help you make and carry out new goals that move you towards a new future (see pages 134 & 138).

8. **Get More Sleep and Rest.** In order to improve your sleep and get more rest (see pages 185-188).
   - *"Day Skills for Night Sleep"*
   - *"Rest in the Bed"*
   - *"Work back to Bed"*

9. **"Look in the Book."** If you recall, on page 207, you learned about a Re-Thinking Skill that improves your memory. By creating a special Memory Book, you will more easily recall appointments and other important information.

10. **Notice Positive Change.** In the days between now and the next Training Week, notice any large or small positive changes that enter your life and write them down. Ask yourself each day:

**"What happened today, large or small,
that I want to see more of in my life?"**

Week Five – Building Positives & the Power of Imagery
Eight Week Basic Training

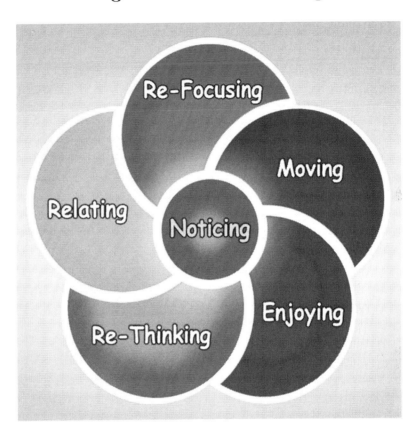

Pain Problems and Comfort Skill Solutions
Included in Week Five

Pain Problems

- *"Attention Hijacked by Pain and Stress"*
- *"Sadness, Worry, & Other Miserable Feelings"*
- *"Hypersensitive Nervous System"*
- *"Distressed by Annoying People*

Comfort Skill Solutions

- *"Go on a Head Trip"*
- *"Counter a Negative with a Positive"*
- *"Write a Gratitude Letter"*
- *"Filling a 'Good Stuff' Journal"*

WEEK FIVE CONTENTS BOX

Making Positive U-Turns
First Training Day

1. The Skill Review
   - A) *"Laughing" or "Doing Fun"*
   - B) *"Breath Massage" or "Immerse in a Good Memory"*
   - C) *"I Want to See More of…"*
2. Today's Pain Problems
   - *Pain Problem #2 - Attention Hijacked by Pain and Stress*
   - *Pain Problem #4 - Sadness Worry, and Other Miserable Feelings*
   - *Pain Problem #6 – Distressed by Annoying People*
3. Learn/About #17 - Making Positive U-Turns
4. Skill of the Day
   - A) *"Counter a Negative with a Positive"*
5. The Last Practice
   - A) *"Immerse in a Good Memory"*
6. Homework Box

Going on a Head Trip
Second Training Day

1. The Skill Review
   - A) Re-Focusing Skill
2. Today's Pain Problems
   - *Pain Problem #2 - Attention Hijacked by Pain and Stress*
   - *Pain Problem #4 - Sadness Worry, and Other Miserable Feelings*
   - *Pain Problem #9 - Hypersensitive Nervous System*
3. Learn/About #18 – Daydreaming on Purpose
4. Skill of the Day (and Last Practice)
   - A) *"The Head Trip"*
5. Homework Box

Cultivating Positive Qualities
Third Training Day

1. The Skill Review
    A) "The Head Trip"
    B) *"I Want to See More of..."*
2. Today's Pain Problems
    ▪ *Pain Problem #4 - Sadness Worry, and Other Miserable Feelings*
    ▪ *Pain Problem #9 - Hypersensitive Nervous System*
3. Learn/About #19 - Cultivating Positive Qualities
4. Skill of the Day
    A) *"Write a Gratitude Letter"*
    B) *"Filling a 'Good Stuff' Journal"*
5. The Last Practice
    A) *"The Head Trip"*
6. Homework Box

Making Positive U-Turns
First Training Day – Week 5

The Skill Review

(A)
Enjoying Skills

Please take a moment and re-read the descriptions of the two Enjoying Skills, "Laughing" and "Doing Fun," and practice at least one of them (see pages 159 & 162).

(B)
Re-Focusing Skills

Practice one of the following Re-Focusing Skills for 20 minutes:
    ▪ *"The Head Trip"* (see page 245)
    ▪ *"Immerse in a Good Memory"* (see page 230)

(C)
"I Want to See More of…"

Consult your Journal or digital file, or review the last several days and answer the two questions below.

- **"What happened since the last Training Day, large or small, that I want to see more of in my life?"**
- **"What caused these things to happen?"**

Today's Pain Problems

Pain Problem #2 – Attention Hijacked by Pain and Stress
Pain Problem #4 – Sadness Worry, and Other Miserable Feelings
Pain Problem #6 – Distressed by Annoying People

Learn/About #17 – Making Positive U-Turns

Often, it is difficult to do something enjoyable when you are hurting or upset. This second Enjoying Skill category offers a way to reverse some of the negativity you face with a strong dose of positivity. Stephanie engaged in a form of this to reduce her work stress.

STORY BOX #25 –
Stephanie Counters Sheila's Negative

Stephanie was a quiet, shy, and very lovely 28-year-old accountant who experienced severe headaches, usually at work. One of her co-workers, Sheila, constantly hassled her about her work load. Stephanie's boss highly valued her work and allowed her to take as many breaks as she needed in order to avoid the headaches.

Sheila didn't care about that and obsessed about Stephanie taking more breaks than her. Never mind the fact that Stephanie felt a 5-7/10 head pain and still managed to do her job. Unfortunately, Sheila's constant nagging and criticism was beginning to push Stephanie's pain level higher and her supervisor could do little to control Sheila's annoying behavior.

In our individual session, Stephanie bemoaned this situation and expressed a sense of hopelessness that she'd ever feel good at work. I told her that she could counter Sheila's negative influence by using what I call

---

the "Double Consequence Solution." After we talked about it, Stephanie became very excited and said that she could hardly wait to use it at work. This Solution is a Relating Skill that not only helps you feel better after a bad encounter with someone like Sheila (first consequence), but it also "punishes" her for annoying you in the first place (second consequence).

The particular Double Consequence method I suggested was something I call "Thanks for the Reminder." The next day, Stephanie had her chance to exercise this Skill by bringing along an interesting novel to work. Once there, she saw Sheila standing by her desk with a scowl on her face. When Stephanie reached her desk, Sheila, as usual, began criticizing her for being "lazy." To that, Stephanie happily responded,

> "Thanks, Sheila, for reminding me that I should take a pre-work break before I start. See ya."

She then walked to the staff room where she sat and read her novel for ten minutes. (Stephanie's boss knew what she was doing this and approved.) In this way, she countered Sheila's Negative (criticism) by engaging in a Positive (reading her book). When Stephanie returned to her desk, she saw Sheila sitting at her desk. As she was about to sit in her chair, Sheila yelled another criticism. Once again, Stephanie joyfully said,

> "Oh, thanks again, Sheila – it's time for another break."

She then sauntered off to the staff room for another ten-minute reading break.

Each time Sheila did or said anything to criticize or pressure her (which was often), Stephanie "thanked" her again and took another unplanned pleasure break. Not only did Stephanie take a number of enjoyable breaks *(First Consequence)*, but when she did she annoyed the heck out of Sheila *(Second Consequence)*. Apparently, Sheila was a little slow in the head and it took her two days to stop criticizing Stephanie.

Stephanie learned that even though Sheila's action upset her, she could dissolve the stress by countering her Negative with a Positive, thus reducing her stress level and headaches and making her job a more peaceful place.

Skill of the Day

"Counter a Negative with a Positive"

This Skill empowers you to reverse some of the harmful effects of a negative experience (Stephanie did one version of this). In another case, a woman I worked with was going through a terrible divorce she told me that every time she had to talk with her soon-to-be-ex-husband, she felt like she needed a bath! In a way, she was right – when you encounter something (or someone) who upsets you, it's as if you just got covered in disgusting, irritating mud. When that happens, it's necessary to wash it off so you'll feel clean and fresh again.[80] This is exactly what the **"Counter a Negative with a Positive"** Skill will do – it clears away some of the distasteful feelings and physical discomfort brought about by distressing situations or annoying people.

ENJOYING SKILL BOX #3 -
"Countering a Negative with a Positive"

Basic Countering.

- *Use Your Fun Menu.* When a person or situation starts to drag you down to a negative place, walk away from them when you can, pull out your Fun Menu, choose one or more enjoyable activities and enjoy them until you feel better.

- *Do a Head Rehearsal.* Sit or lie down and imagine you're in a painful or upsetting situation. Next, picture yourself walking away from it, looking at your Fun Menu, and picking something good to do. Example – One woman imagined that she walked away from an annoying argument with a criticizing family member. Next, she imagined going out for a drive along the beach, then taking herself out to dinner. (She eventually did this activity and felt a whole lot better.)

Targeted Countering

- **Positive Scoring.** If you want, you can use a one-to-ten scale and assign a number to each item on your Fun Menu that corresponds to how good it makes you feel. Example - "listening to a good song" as a 4/10 positive event, or score "seeing a movie" as an 8/10 positive.

---

[80] This is true inside your body since a stressful encounter can physically flood you with stress hormones that "muddy up" your system and contribute to discomfort and other health problems.

> - **Targeted Countering**. When you're faced with a negative person or situation, walk away to a safe place. Once you get there, consider how bad your encounter was and score it. Finally, counter it with a higher Positive on your Fun Menu. Example – A man in pain was unreasonably criticized by his wife for being "lazy." After he walked away from her, he noticed that he felt a 7/10 Negative (depressed). Looking at his Menu, he chose an 8/10 Positive (going out to a movie and a delicious dinner). Doing this cleaned away a lot of his wife's criticism and his mood improved.

Take some time now and consider how you would practice this Skill in negative situations you've experienced.

The Last Practice
"Immerse in a Good Memory"
Practice this Re-Focusing Skill for 20 minutes (see page 230).

HOMEWORK BOX
FIRST TRAINING DAY – WEEK 5

1. **Practice Any Re-Focusing Skill.** Each day, for at least 20 minutes, practice one or more of Re-Focusing Skills #'s 1-5 (see list on page 338).

2. **Enjoy Yourself NOW!** Use "Laughter" and "Doing Fun" to bring more pleasure into your life. Do something enjoyable at least five times a week (see pages 159 & 163).

3. **Positive U-Turn Rehearsal.** Recall one or more difficult situations from your past and imagine how you would use the *"Counter a Negative with a Positive"* Skill to make a Positive U-Turn (see Box above).

4. **Notice Positive Change.** In the days between now and the next Training Day, notice any large or small positive changes that enter your life and write them down. Ask yourself each day:

> **"What happened today, large or small,**
> **that I want to see more of in my life?"**

Go on a Head Trip
Second Training Day – Week 5

The Skill Review

(A)
Re-Focusing Skill

For 20 minutes, practice one of the first four Re-Focusing Skills listed on page 338.

(B)
"I Want to See More of…"

Consult your Journal or digital file, or memory and answer the two questions below.

- **"What happened since the last Training Day, large or small, that I want to see more of in my life?"**
- **"What caused these things to happen?"**

Today's Pain Problems

Pain Problem #2 – Attention Hijacked by Pain and Stress
Pain Problem #4 – Sadness Worry, and Other Miserable Feelings
Pain Problem #9 – Hypersensitive Nervous System

Learn/About #18 – Day Dreaming on Purpose

When we use our imagination, it's like we're "daydreaming on purpose." **"Daydreaming on Purpose"** *is the intentional use of your imagination to have a desired experience.* Often, you can choose to go somewhere and/or do something in your mind that you can't ordinarily do in the real world. This often causes you to feel like you've actually visited your chosen destination or experience. Some of you may see, hear, or feel things in your imagination – all of these come in handy when you want to get a little relief from Misery.

Remember the times when you sat in a boring high school or college class or some kind of a meeting and you found your mind wandering to more interesting places. In other words, you were able to temporarily escape from the boredom by daydreaming. Perhaps you've also done this while sitting or lying down on a couch or in bed. For some of you, the doctor's waiting room is a popular place to let your attention drift away to dreamy places. You might imagine taking an enjoyable trip, eating a great meal, kissing someone you love, and even replaying a great movie in your head. When you "Daydream on Purpose," you might feel as if you're temporarily leaving your body and traveling to a beautiful, faraway place. This is the power of your imagination.

The Beach in Three Senses.

Like in daydreaming, you can use your five senses to see, hear, feel, taste, or smell anything in your mind. However, most people will tend to emphasize one or two senses over the others. For example, let's say that you want to imagine that you're at the beach on a sunny Summer afternoon. Typically, many of you will use one of three dominant senses: seeing, hearing, or feeling. If you have a well-developed visual ability, you'll imagine the beach in your mind's eye – seeing the sun and the waves and the white sands and the blue water. If you have a strong ear, you'll hear the waves and the light wind blowing in your ears; you'll hear kids playing on the beach or hear the calls of the seagulls. If you feel deeply, you may sense the warm sun on your body as you lie on soft towel, or imagine digging your hands into the sand feeling the cool sensation, or picturing yourself walking along the shore and feeling your feet wading through warm water. Finally, some of you can experience this imaginary beach through a mix of those sensations. Overall, daydreaming on purpose can relax your body, distract your mind, raise your mood, and increase your Comfort.

The next two Boxes will provide examples of some of the daydreams that my clients have purposely created. Following that, you can learn how to create some of your own.

STORY BOX #26 –
Stan's Dripping Feet

Stan's is a 62-year-old gentleman suffering from Neuropathic pain in both of his feet. A former part-time preacher, he felt that G-d had abandoned him to a life of pain, despair, and hopelessness. He stopped going to church. When Stan came to my Comfort Workshop, he felt suicidal, angry, and depressed, and he told us that he was at the end of his rope. The people in the Workshop were able to give him a lot of support and soon he started to benefit from practicing some of the Comfort Strategies.

At one session, I invited people to picture the pain as some recognizable substance filling up the afflicted part of their body. Then I asked them to imagine fading it out of their bodies.

After we finished the exercise, Stan was smiling! When I asked the members of the group to talk about their experience, Stan's hand shot up and he immediately, and very excitedly, began to tell us what happened. He said that he felt 200% more comfortable! He told us that he'd always imagined his feet felt like they were filled with "fiery red chemicals" that burned and burned no matter what he tried to do to stop the pain. In the exercise, he imagined seeing the pain as that red liquid concentrated in the bottoms of his feet and toes. Then, he became curious to find out what would happen if he imagined little holes opening up in his toes.

In his mind's eye, he saw the painful red stuff dripping hot drops out of these imagined holes onto the floor and the carpet absorbed them. To his surprise, Stan said that when this happened, he noticed a slow easing of the pain in his feet. After the 20-minute exercises ended, he discovered that he drained all the fiery chemicals out of his body and he felt great.

Although this effect only lasted 15 minutes, Stan practiced it diligently for months after the Workshop ended. He called me one day and said that although the condition was still there, it was easier for him to control it for longer periods of time using his imagination and other Skills. The last time I spoke with him, he had become active in a new church community.

STORY BOX #27 –
Stacey's Butt Faucet

Stacey is a 32-year-old mother of three who unfortunately hurt her low back in a skiing accident. By the time I met her, she had endured three years of pain, gaining little help from the medical-only treatments she'd received. She was in bed a lot and felt bad that she could not be the mother or wife she wanted to be for her family. Her doctor eventually sent her to the pain program.

She got a lot out of the Comfort Skills Workshop and went on to join my Re-Focusing Skills group. In this special workshop, members learned a number of practices that they used to increase their body Comfort. At the end of one Imagery session, Stacey was smiling like an idiot and told us this:

> "I imagined that I stuck a faucet end into my butt cheek and when I opened the spout, a stream of muddy gunk came pouring out. As I saw this happen, I noticed that the reservoir of pain in my low back and butt was emptying and before we finished the Imagery session it was mostly gone!"

Later, Stacey told us that she practiced her "butt faucet imagery" often and it enabled her to do more at home. She also felt a little more like the person she used to be.

Skill of the Day (and Last Practice)

"The Head Trip"

How would you like to go anywhere you want in (or out) of this world absolutely free? How about going to fascinating places or traveling back in time? You can go to Tahiti, Italy, Morocco, the North Pole, visit Harry Potter's Hogwarts School, or the moon. You can ride around with 19th Century Texas Rangers, talk with Jane Austen or Albert Einstein, fight Samurai warriors, play ball with your favorite team, or even hang out in the court of a French or Hawaiian King. Imagine that you could do anything you wanted in these or other places and eras. Even better, you can have any kind of body, one that has no limits or disabilities. All of this can happen when you go on a "Head Trip," which is simply imagining that you are going on a trip in your head. The only down-side of this Skill is that you won't get any travel miles for your trip! Although you can't bring back gifts, you may return with a comfortable feeling. Try this method to "Daydream on Purpose."

FOCUSING SKILL BOX #5 – "The Head Trip"

Step One - Quiet Place and Timer. Sit in a comfortable seat in a quiet place and set your timer for twenty-minutes.

Step Two - Choose a Trip. When you're ready, think about a place or historical time you'd like to visit or an experience you'd like to have. You can keep a list of your favorite places to daydream in your Journal or digital file.

Step Three – Four Trip Qualities. On your trip, you can choose to:
1) *Go anywhere you want* (i.e., Hawaii beaches or in a sailboat with your grandfather).
2) *Do whatever you'd like to do there* (i.e., climb a mountain).
3) *Bring guests or go alone* (i.e., you and your little sister go out on the town).
4) *Have any kind of a body you'd like to have* (a big, strong body that can climb mountains).

Step Four – Now Take the Trip. Once you've chosen your Trip, allow yourself to travel there any way you'd like. Suggestions include:

- *Count Yourself There.* Count from ten down to one, and imagine that you appear at your destination once you reach "one."
- *Start with Clothes.* Imagine that you're in your bedroom standing in your underwear. Begin to dress in the clothes that you'll need to wear in the place you're going. Once you're all dressed, you'll be there.
- *Get a Vehicle.* See yourself getting onto some means of transportation (i.e. a jet or boat) that takes you to the place you want to visit.

Step Five - Returning. Once you are ready to return to the room, use any method you'd like (i.e., number count from "one" up to "ten").

Remember

- ➤ *Distractions.* Once you begin your trip, enjoy yourself. If you get distracted by anything, just let it go and return to your trip.
- ➤ *Control.* You are in complete control of this experience and can change it at any time.
- ➤ *Bodily Adjustments.* Know that you can adjust your body for comfort any time and then return back to your trip.
- ➤ *"Interference Thought"* **WARNING!!** Sometimes, as you are imagining yourself in interesting places doing enjoyable activities, you may get an uninvited thought that screams something like, ***"OH YEAH!? –I CAN'T DO THAT ANYMORE!!*** Treat these *"Interference Thoughts"* like any other Negative Thoughts – notice them and let them go. Then, return to focusing on your Trip.

Okay, now use the Skill Box above to sit for a period of time and practice the "Head Trip."

HOMEWORK BOX
SECOND TRAINING DAY – WEEK 5

1. **Go on "The Head Trip.".** For 20 minutes, practice this Skill once a day until the next Training Day (see above Box).

2. **Practice Enjoying Now!** For three times this week, practice an Enjoying Skill to bring more pleasure into your life (see page 158 & 163).

3. **Positive U-Turn Rehearsal.** Recall one or more difficult situations from your past and imagine how you would use the "Counter a Negative with a Positive" Skill to make a Positive U-Turn (see page 239).

4. **Notice Positive Change.** In the days between now and the next Training Day, notice any large or small positive changes that enter your life and write them down. Ask yourself each day:

   "What happened today, large or small,
   that I want to see more of in my life?"

Cultivating Positive Qualities
Third Training Day – Week 5

The Skill Review

(A)
"The Head Trip"

Practice this Re-Focusing Skill for at least 20 minutes (see page 245).

(B)
"I Want to See More of…"

Consult your Journal or digital file, or review the last several days and answer the two questions below.

- "What happened since the last Training Day, large or small, that I want to see more of in my life?"
- "What caused these things to happen?"

Today's Pain Problem
Pain Problem #4 – Sadness Worry, and Other Miserable Feelings

Learn/About #19 – Cultivating Positive Qualities

A third category of Enjoying Skills develops your "Positive Qualities." A **"Positive Quality"** *is a strongly held, life affirming purpose, meaning, value, and/or ability that defines your character*. It uplifts your spirit and has a constructive impact on the world around you.

Research shows that when you cultivate generosity, love of learning, humor, spirituality, or any of twenty other Qualities, your well-being can increase. For example, if you hold the Positive Quality of "Curiosity," you're the kind of person who is fascinated with people, places, ideas, and/or things. You love exploring their characteristics and differences and you get excited when you discover these. This may include tasting various foods, listening to a new type of music, or even noticing how various Comfort Skills affect your body. Some of your acts of Curiosity (i.e., asking questions) may stimulate the interest of the people around you. It can also move your mind (and nervous system) away from discomfort and towards something more fun.

These Qualities have been studied by a number of scientists over the years.[81] Most recently, the Positive psychologists Christopher Peterson and Martin Seligman identified twenty-four "Signature Strengths." They observed that people experience these in several ways:

1. Gaining a sense of Quality ownership and realizing that it's who they "really are"
2. Getting excited when they exercise them
3. Feeling motivated to act in ways that reflect the Qualities
4. Using them effectively and adapting them to new situations very quickly
5. Feeling energized and invigorated rather than exhausted by them[82]

---

[81] See the 1937 book by Gordon Allport entitled, "Personality: A psychological interpretation."

[82] See "Character Strengths and Virtues: A Handbook and Classification," by Christopher Peterson and Martin Seligman, 2004; also see "Primer in Positive Psychology," by Christopher Peterson, 2006.

Cultivating Positive Qualities

For centuries, different cultures, religious traditions, and philosophies have promoted the exercise of positive character traits and personal values. More recently, scientists who study personal values and character strengths have found that as you practice your Positive Qualities, they will improve your life. In one specific study, researchers discovered that individuals who expanded on their Quality in new ways were able to reduce depression better than the best known psychological treatment for depression, Cognitive-Behavioral Therapy.[83]

STORY BOX #28 –
Sophee the Pain Comedian

Sophee used to love comedy. But when she was injured in a motorcycle accident, the resulting leg pain overwhelmed her with depression and misery. At 29 years of age, she was already anticipating a terrible future and this caused her to become absorbed in the sad thought that pain and disappointment were all she could look forward to. She also felt stressed out by the fact that she had no savings and soon her disability money would run out. Desperately, she tried to find jobs that wouldn't turn on the chronic pain in her left leg. None were found.

The answer came on a good day while she was visiting her sister and some friends. Sometime during their get-together, Sophee made a funny comment and immediately the whole group screamed out a roar of laughter. This made her laugh a little. When she made another joke, they laughed again. Soon, she found herself making more funny statements, one after the other, which caused the little gathering of women to rock back and forth in waves of laughter.

Later, at home, while she was icing her leg, Sophee thought deeply and fondly about that incident. It occurred to her that she felt very natural and comfortable getting people to laugh and this reminded her of her high school days when she used to do amateur stand-up comedy routines in school performances. What was really interesting is that as she thought about those days she felt better.

---

[83] See a 2005 article by Martin Seligman and his colleagues entitled, "Positive psychology progress: Empirical validation of interventions" in the journal, American Psychologist (pages 410-421).

> When we met in a session the next day, I talked with her about the positive effects that come from developing one's Positive Qualities and that it looked like she had the Quality of Humor. Not only did she love to laugh, but she excelled at getting other people to laugh. So we talked about how she could develop it further. She decided to build up her humor muscle by first watching her favorite comedians every day. She used a combination of YouTube, TV, DVDs, and, occasionally, she went to comedy clubs with her friends. Next, she put together a few routines and performed them at a local comedy club during its "open mike night." She eventually developed her own style, which distinguished her from other comics. In time, she became very popular and the club owner hired her as a regular.
>
> Sophee performed both "stand-up" and "sit down" comedy so she could rest her leg. A year later, she was working part-time on a comedy circuit that included night clubs, parties, and other events. At the same time that her Quality of Humor gave others a great deal of belly laughs, it also gave her a meaningful, part-time job and a sense of accomplishment and purpose.

Positive Quality List

Although you probably know some of your Positive Qualities, you'll still find it useful to explore new ones. A number of cultures, religions, and social theories include collections of these.[84] As mentioned above, one such list of Qualities was created by Positive Psychologist Christopher Peterson and his colleagues. They compiled a well-researched set of what they call "Signature Strengths." There are twenty-four of them grouped under 6 categories.[85] In the following Info Box, I've listed these and their brief descriptions.

Following these Boxes, we will focus on the development of one particular Quality that can help people-in-pain eventually feel "bigger than the pain." This Quality is called "Gratitude."

---

[84] A brief set of Quality lists from other traditions are included on the following websites:
Judaism - http://www.c-bh.com/pages/midot.htm
Christianity - http://www.discipleshiptools.org/apps/articles/default.asp?articleid=37084&columnid=4166
Muslim - http://www.islamondemand.com/islamic_virtues.html
Humanist - http://www.virtuescience.com/virtuelist.html
[85] See http://www.viacharacter.org/PRACTICE/Exercisestobuildyourcharacterstrengths.aspx and click on the "VIA Classification of character Strengths on http://wwwthehappinessinstitute.com. Signature Strengths Info.

INFO BOX #23 -
POSITIVE QUALITIES
("Strengths")

Wisdom and Knowledge
(These involve the acquisition and use of knowledge)

1. **Creativity**. Thinking of novel and productive ways to conceptualize and do things.
2. **Curiosity**. Taking an interest in ongoing experience for its own sake; exploring new things.
3. **Open-Mindedness.** Looking at things from all sides; weighing all evidence fairly.
4. **Love of Learning.** Mastering new skills, subjects, & knowledge.
5. **Wise Perspective.** Giving wise counsel to people; making sense of life for oneself and others.

Courage
(These involve using personal will to surmount obstacles)

6. **Bravery**. Meeting threat, challenge, difficulty, or pain with courage; acting on beliefs even if they're unpopular.
7. **Perseverance.** Sticking with what you started and persisting in a course of action in spite of obstacles.
8. **Integrity**. Presenting oneself in a genuine way; taking responsibility for one's feeling and actions.
9. **Vitality**. Approaching life with excitement and energy; feeling alive and activated.

Humanity
(These involve helping and befriending other people)

10. **Love**. Valuing close relations with others where sharing and caring are mutually exchanged. \
11. **Kindness**. Doing favors and good deeds for others; being nice.
12. **Emotional Intelligence**. Being aware of motives and feelings of other people and oneself.

Justice
(These promote communal and universal values)

13. **Social Responsibility.** Working well as a member of a group or team; being loyal to the group.
14. **Fairness.** Treating all people equally based on fundamental fairness without personal bias.
15. **Leadership.** Directing one's group in accomplishing a goal and maintaining their good relations.

Discipline
(These protect you against personal excess)

16. **Forgiveness and Mercy.** Forgiving people, accepting their shortcomings, giving second chances.
17. **Humility.** Letting one's accomplishments speak for themselves; not regarding oneself as too special.
18. **Moderation.** Careful about one's choices; avoiding unnecessary risks and things that may cause regret.
19. **Self-Control.** Regulating what one feels and does; being disciplined in action, appetite, and emotion.
20. **Bravery.** Meeting threat, challenge, difficulty, or pain; acting on beliefs even if they are unpopular.

Expansiveness
*(These reveal connections to a
larger universe of meaning)*

21. **Hope.** Optimistically looking towards the future and working to achieve the best outcome possible.
22. **Humor.** Being playful, laughing easily, bringing smiles to other people; seeing the light side.
23. **Spirituality.** Having solid beliefs about and deep experiences of a higher purpose and meaning of life.
24. **Gratitude.** Being aware of and thankful for the good things that happen; expressing thanks.

Skills of the Day

Gratitude – A Brief Introduction

When you cultivate your Positive Qualities, you enhance your ability to improve your mood and create a happier and more satisfying life.[86] You also strengthen your physical comfort. A full description of how to develop each of these Qualities is beyond the scope of this book; however, the two Skills offered below show how you can explore one of them: **"Gratitude,"** *is a Positive Quality that fills your heart with feelings of appreciation and thankfulness*. It's one of the most commonly held Positive Qualities. [87] According to a study that looked at twenty-four Signature Strengths, most people identified Gratitude as one of the top five Qualities that they labeled "most like me."[88]

Use the Gratitude Skills to increase your sense of appreciation and personal meaning. Over time, your Quality of Gratitude will grow into a powerful deterrent to hopelessness, despair and the other Negatives that often accompany chronic pain. It'll also raise your awareness of the good that surrounds you each moment of your day (although at first, this may seem impossible). Finally, Gratitude helps you to remember and appreciate past positive events and people.

(A)
"Write a Gratitude Letter"

When you express Gratitude, you stimulate positive, health-building emotions in yourself and in other people.

ENJOYING SKILL BOX #4 -
"Write a Gratitude Letter"

Step One - Choose a Person or Situation. Search your memory and recall people or moments in your life that gave you deep feelings of appreciation. Maybe they did something wonderful for you or you just felt grateful for their presence in your life.

---

[86] "The How of Happiness" by Sonja Lyubimirsky.

[87] Learn how to develop other qualities on that list by consulting the following sources: a) A book by Christopher Peterson and Martin Seligman, "Character Strengths and Virtues," 2004; b) The article, "Want to Feel Happier? A Menu of Resolutions" by Gretchen Rubin. Also search online for "List of 24 Signature Strengths;" c) "Thanks" by Robert A Emmons.

[88] See Nansook Park, Christopher Peterson, and Martin Seligman in their 2006 article, "Character Strengths in 54 Nations and All 50 U.S. States," 2006.

Step Two - Write Them a Letter. Write a one-page letter to that person describing what you're grateful for. Here are some suggestions:
   A) *What Happened?* Be very detailed in this note. What did the person do and how did it affect your life? How did their actions make you feel and what did you learn from them?
   B) *General Appreciation.* If the letter is for someone you genuinely appreciate, list at least three specific positive things you love about them.
   C) *Make it Permanent.* Since you'll give this letter to the person, laminate or frame it so it will last for a long time. (If it's about a person who is deceased, imagine reading it to them.)

Step Three – Go on a "Gratitude Date." Choose a time to meet with the person and read them the letter. It's best to do this in person and not on the phone. Perhaps you can take them out to lunch or go to a beautiful place. Give yourself enough time to be together to exchange thoughts and feelings about the letter.

(B)

"Filling a Good Stuff Journal"

Too often, Depression and other Bad Guys convince you to forget the good in your life. One powerful means of countering this is to take a little time each day to write down what you feel grateful for. This will increase the strength of those blessings. When this exercise becomes second nature, it'll strengthen your Quality of Gratitude and raise your level of joy.

ENJOYING SKILL BOX #5 –
"Filling a Good Stuff Journal"

Step One - Get a Blank Journal. Acquire a blank journal or use a digital file. Get one of these and give it a name (i.e., "Good Stuff Journal").

Step Two - Choose a Time and Place. Choose a time and place towards the end of the day when you're free to sit or lie comfortably and write in your journal. It's useful to pick two times and places to do this writing so that if you miss the first, you can do the second (i.e., right after dinner while sitting in your easy chair or by your bedside just before sleep).

Step Three - Record Good Stuff in Your Journal.
- *Choose Three.* Although it may be a challenge, do your best to record at least three recent events that you feel grateful for.
- *Repeaters.* If your list starts becoming repetitive, break down the benefits into multiple parts and reflect on each separately. For example, if you're grateful for the meals your spouse makes for you, consider something different that you like in each meal (i.e., the flavor of the roasted chicken or the texture of a pudding dessert).

Step Four - Read What You Got. Once you've collected some of these grateful moments, take some time each week to read them. Let them inspire you to greater appreciation for the good things you have. For example, you might decide to read your Journal during Sunday lunch.

The Last Practice
"The Head Trip"

Use this Skill to take yourself on a little adventure in your head. Engage in it for at least twenty minutes right now (see page 245).

HOMEWORK BOX
THIRD TRAINING DAY – WEEK 5

1. **Go On "The Head Trip."** Use this Re-Focusing Skill to take a well-deserved vacation in your mind. Do it for at least 20 minutes each day (see page 245).

2. **Practice the Gratitude Skills.** Use the steps in the Skill Boxes above.

3. **Positive U-Turn Rehearsal.** Recall one or more difficult situations from your past and imagine how you would use the *"Counter a Negative with a Positive"* Skill to make a Positive U-Turn (see page 239).

4. **Notice Positive Change.** In the days between now and the next Training Day, notice any large or small positive changes that enter your life and write them down. Ask yourself each day:

    "What happened today, large or small, that I want to see more of in my life?"

Week Six – Meeting Good People & Flare Planning
Eight Week Basic Training

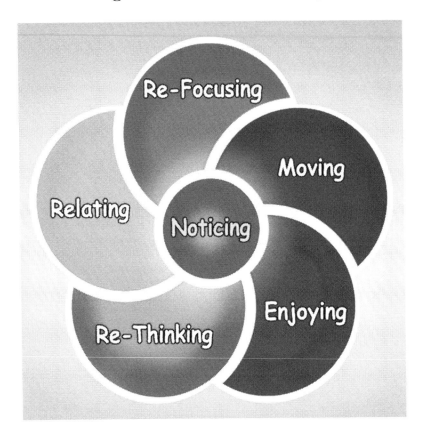

Pain Problems and Comfort Skill Solutions Included in Week Six

Pain Problems

- *"Attention Hijacked by Pain and Stress"*
- *"Sadness, Worry, & Other Miserable Feelings"*
- *"Hypersensitive Nervous System"*
- *"Isolation and Loneliness"*
- *"Underprepared for Pain Flares"*

Comfort Skill Solutions

- *"Build New Relationships with Old Friends and Family"*
- *"How to Meet New Friends"*
- *"Positive Distraction – The Fast and Slow Menus"*
- *"Flare Planning in Sets of Three"*
- *"Two Bottles of Comfort"*

WEEK SIX CONTENTS BOX

Relating with Good People
First Training Day

1. The Skill Review
   A) Re-Focusing Skills
   B) *"I want to See More of..."*
2. Today's Pain Problem
   - *Pain Problem #13 – Isolation and Loneliness*
3. Learn/About #20 – The Relating Strategy and Relating with Good People
4. Skills of the Day
   A) *"Build New Relationships with Old Friends and Family"*
   B) *"How to Meet New Friends"*
5. The Last Practice
   A) Re-Focusing Skills
6. Homework Box

Positive Distractions
Second Training Day

1. The Skill Review
   A) Re-Focusing Skills
   B) *"I want to See More of..."*
2. Today's Pain Problems
   - *Pain Problem #2 - Attention Hijacked by Pain and Stress*
   - *Pain Problem #4 - Sadness Worry, and Other Miserable Feelings*
   - *Pain Problem #9 - Hypersensitive Nervous System*
3. Skill of the Day
   A) *"Positive Distraction - The Fast and Slow Menus"*
4. The Last Practice
   A) Re-Focusing Skills
5. Homework Box

Flare Planning
Third Training Day

1. The Skill Review
   A) Re-Focusing Skills
   B) *"I want to See More of..."*
2. Today's Pain Problem
   - *Pain Problem #7 - Underprepared for Pain Flares*
3. Skills of the Day
   A) *"Flare Planning in Sets of Three"*
   B) *"Two Bottles of Comfort"*
4. The Last Practice
   A) Re-Focusing Skills
5. Homework Box

Relating with Good People
First Training Day – Week 6

The Skill Review

(A)
Re-Focusing Skills

Practice one of the following Re-Focusing Skills for 20 minutes:
   - *"The Head Trip"* (see page 245)
   - *"Immerse in a Good Memory"* (see page 230)

(B)
"I Want to See More of..."

Review your Journal or digital file and answer these questions:
   - "What happened since the last Training Day, large or small, that I want to see more of in my life?"
   - "What caused these things to happen?"

Today's Pain Problem
Pain Problem #13 – Isolation and Loneliness

Learn/About #20 –
The Relating Strategy & Relating with Good People

The **"Relating Strategy"** *empowers you to both increase your positive connections to people and set limits on those who annoy you.* We all relate – with ourselves, with people, with the environment and, for some of us, with our Spiritual Source. One definition of the word "relating" is "connecting with someone." Skills in this Strategy empower you to revive your previous social life and create new relationships. There is a growing body of research that suggests that building a positive social life improves your physical and emotional health.[89]

Relationships are wonderful to develop and grow. However, they also can also be challenging and frustrating. It is important to get closer to people you know and to connect with and family and friends when these relationships are mutually respectful. As many of you know, when people treat you badly, the pain is likely to rise. When that happens, you can make your way back to Comfort by setting limits on their bad behavior. In the Week Seven trainings, you'll learn about "Annoying People" and how to set limits on them.

In the sections below, you will learn Relating Skills that help you to leave loneliness behind by pursuing relationships with good people.

Skills of the Day

(A)
"Build New Relationships with Old Friends and Family"

Many people-in-pain become socially isolated. This is because (i) they either don't feel comfortable around others, and/or (ii) they were abandoned by some of their family and friends. Despite this, it's very possible to rekindle a social life. When you connect with good people by sharing pleasurable activities, talking, laughing, and solving problems together, you benefit with increased support, health, and Comfort. Whether you are having good times with friends, hanging out with family, or chatting with a friendly co-worker – positive social time that does not overly strain your body will distract you and enhance your relief and quality of life.

---

[89] See "Love and Survival: Eight Pathways to Intimacy and Health" by Dean Ornish.

RELATING SKILL BOX #1 -
"Build New Relationships with Old Friends and Family"

Step One - Make a List of Old Friends & Family You'd Like to Spend Time With. This first, small step is fairly easy to do and requires little commitment on your part. Take your time in building the list and review it from time to time. Perhaps you'll decide to remove some names or add others.

Step Two – Re-Connect with People. Here are four ways to re-connect with family and old friends.

- *Make Phone Dates.* Connect on the phone. For those of you either home-bound or not ready to meet face-to-face, a telephone conversation is a good first meeting place because it allows you to control the length of your conversation. It also allows you to gauge whether or not you want more contact with the person in the future.

- *Invite Someone to Visit You at Home.* If you want to visit with someone, but you're not ready to go out, set up visit times in your home. Perhaps you'll decide to do something fun, like playing cards or video games, watching a movie, or dinner. By doing this, you also learn how much the person wants to be with you - if they like spending time with you on your turf, perhaps this means that they enjoy your company. (People-in-pain often find that some of their "friends" only want to spend time with them around specific events, like skiing or hiking.)

- *Go Out with Old Friends and Family.* When you're ready to spend time with people outside of your home, set up an outing. Make sure it's doable and plan to engage in it for a comfortable amount of time. For example – If you plan to go out to dinner, make sure that beforehand you discuss with the person your physical limitations and allow the possibility that you may have to cut dinner short, if necessary. Should that happen you can make a "Plan B" if you want to continue spending time with them (i.e., go home and watch a film together).

> - *Host a Gathering.* A party night sounds good, but it may also sound like a lot of work. It won't be if you organize it with others. Example - If you want to host a meal, avoid cooking by holding it in a nearby restaurant or inviting people to bring pot-luck. Let your loved ones do most of the setting up and cleaning up. This will lower your stress level and prevent pain flares. In the end, you'll enjoy the presence of a supportive community of family and friends.

Okay, now take some time now and consider one person in your family, or an old friend, who you would like to spend time with. Use some of the ideas in the Skill Box above to plan how you can renew or strengthen your relationship with them.

(B)
"How to Meet New Friends"

Some of you may not have anyone in your life to connect with. Try the following.

RELATING SKILL BOX #2 -
"How to Meet New Friends"

Step One - Make a List of Your Personal Qualities. We usually like to spend time with people who hold some or most of our values, beliefs, and ideals. Perhaps you like folks who are generous or funny. Write these down and create a profile of what potential friends would look like. As you meet new people, you'll become aware of those who share your Qualities. For example, if you have the Quality of Humor, you'll choose to spend time with people who laugh and joke easily.

Step Two - Make a List of Your Interests. "Interests" are activities and subjects that you like to pursue. Interesting subject areas may include religion, spirituality, politics, sports, food, camping, etc. Examples of specific activities may include 1) attending Church, 2) sitting with a meditation group, 3) attending a baseball game, or 4) going to a ball game or concert. Your interests can guide you in your selection of social groups as well. For example, if you're the kind of person who loves to read novels and discuss them, you might decide to read a novel with someone or join a book club.

Step Three – Begin to Identify and Explore Individuals or Groups that Share Your Personal Qualities and Interests.

Explore social possibilities by consulting with friends, using a phone book, or surfing the Internet. You may want to explore some of these sources:

A) Religious or spiritual communities
B) Science, computer, or nature societies
C) Social media and Internet-based groups
D) Book clubs and other activity groups (i.e., hiking)
E) Community College or Adult-School classes
F) Political parties or social action organizations
G) Volunteer agencies (i.e., at hospitals or schools)
H) Theater, musical, or dance performance groups
I) Social parties, concerts, fairs and festivals

Step Four – Visit Some of These Places & People or Join Those You Like. When you're ready, select one or two individuals or groups and spend time with them. In this way, you can "taste-test" the people and the activities. If they fit you, spend more time with them. Some of you might decide to join an organization.

Remember

You don't have to rush. Give yourself permission to take Baby Steps towards building a new social life.

The Last Practice
Re-Focusing Skills

Practice one of the following Re-Focusing Skills for 20 minutes.

- *"The Head Trip"* (page 245)
- *"Immerse in a Good Memory"* (page 230)

HOMEWORK BOX
FIRST TRAINING DAY – WEEK 6

1. **Practice "The Head Trip" or "Immerse in a Good Memory."** Use one of these Re-Focusing Skills for at least twenty minutes each day (page 245 or 230).

2. **Build Social Connections.** Take a few Baby Steps towards spending time with good people. If you already do this, do a little more. Use the two Relating Skill Boxes above to help you connect.

3. **Notice Positive Change.** In the days between now and the next Training Day, notice any large or small positive changes that enter your life and write them down. Ask yourself each day:

> "What happened today, large or small,
> that I want to see more of in my life?"

Positive Distractions
Second Training Day – Week 6

The Skill Review

(A)
Re-Focusing Skills

Practice one of the following Re-Focusing Skills for 20 minutes (see Chapter Three for location of instructions).

- *"The Head Trip"* (page 245)
- *"Immerse in a Good Memory"* (page 230)

(B)
"I Want to See More of…"

Consult your Journal, or review the last several days and answer the two questions below.

- **"What happened since the last Training Day, large or small, that I want to see more of in my life?"**
- **"What caused these things to happen?"**

Today's Pain Problem

Pain Problem #2 – Attention is Hijacked by Pain and Stress
Pain Problem #4 – Sadness Worry, and Other Miserable Feelings
Pain Problem #9 – Hypersensitive Nervous System

Skill of the Day

Positive Distraction – An Introduction

"Positive Distractions" *are activities and events that positively engage your attention.* Examples include working on a project that you want to complete, finishing your housework, taking a walk, or doing an errand. These may not be as enjoyable as "Doing Fun" (see page 162), but they temporarily draw your attention away from the pain and redirect it elsewhere. As you do this, your attention settles less on chronic pain and more on Comfort.

STORY BOX #29 – Billy's African Adventure

Billy felt cooped up in his apartment ever since he realized that his low back condition was going to be there "forever." He was injured in a car crash while working as a police officer. Living on disability, he'd been moping around the house for months. Billy was in his thirties and he really wanted to get out and <u>do</u> something, but he feared the pain. Finally, the day came when he decided to do something to stop chronic pain from keeping him stuck in the house.

I was shocked and surprised when he told me what he did. Billy said that he was "sick and tired of being sick and tired" and that he realized that whether he was inside his apartment lying around or outside doing some moderate activity, he was still going to hurt. In light of this, he decided that he wanted to do something interesting while he hurt. This led him to drive to a local wild animal park and go on one of their tours - he was driven around an open zoo park and saw African animals wandering about freely.

Even though Billy was bouncing around in that vehicle, he had a great time. He said that a giraffe came up to their parked vehicle and began chewing on the fabric roof! He told me that even though the pain level did not change a great deal, the distractions kept his mind happily busy. He took many great pictures and later he invited friends over for a slide-show.

After that, he realized that his increased mood and feeling of accomplishment also served to increase his Comfort level.

(A)
"Positive Distraction – The Fast and Slow Menus"

You probably do a number of things to distract your mind from Pain, including watching funny movies, doing your bills, eating something good, or even sitting in your backyard. You can create a menu of these activities and other diversions by writing them down in one place, perhaps in a journal. You can look at your "Positive Distraction Menu" and choose from any of its selections. The next Skill Box suggests two different types of Distraction Menus.

RE-FOCUSING SKILL BOX #7 -
"Positive Distraction – The Fast and Slow Menus"

The Fast Distraction Menu

Step One - Settle in with Your Materials. Get your Journal or a digital file and settle yourself into a comfortable place.

Step Two – Fast Distraction. You can do these right away for a brief or medium period of time. Search your memory and recall at least ten to twenty distractions that you can use quickly and easily without increasing the pain. Although these are activities that you can plan and begin doing within an hour, you can engage in them as long as you'd like. For example, sitting in a lounge chair by your garden and looking at your plants, or watching the clouds from a window in your house, or even washing your dishes (if you can do it comfortably).

Step Three - Make a Menu. Write them down on your own Fast Distraction Menu and keep it with you wherever you go.

Step Four - Using the Fast Menu. Pull out your Fast Menu when you need a quick distraction and do one or more on your list.

The Slow Distraction Menu

Step One - Settle in with Your Materials. Get your Journal or a digital file and settle yourself into a comfortable place.

Step Two – Slow Distraction. These distractions need more preparation time and may last longer. Search your memory and recall at least ten to twenty, medium-sized or large distractions that you can do within a several hours to several days. They often include tasks you need to complete. Example – carefully organizing a corner of your garage, cooking a nice dinner, shopping at a distant store, or sit at the beach and people-watch.

Step Three - Make a Menu. Write them down in your Journal or on a digital file and keep it with you wherever you go.

Step Four - Using the Slow Distraction Menu. Pull out this Menu and select an activity from the list that will give you a longer-lasting distraction. Give yourself time to prepare for it.

Okay, now take some time and create a "Fast" and "Slow" Menu and plan to use at least one of them within the next couple of days.

The Last Practice
Re-Focusing Skills

For 20 minutes, practice Re-Focusing Skills #'s 1-5 or 7-8 found listed on page 338.

HOMEWORK BOX
SECOND TRAINING DAY – WEEK 6

1. **Practice "The Head Trip."** Use this Focusing Skill to take yourself on a well-deserved vacation. Do it for at least twenty minutes each day between now and the next Training Day (see page 245).

2. **Build Social Connections.** Take a few more steps towards spending time with people. If you already do this, do a little more. Use the first two Relating Skill Boxes to help you do this (see pages 260-262).

3. **Make a Positive Distraction Menu.** Create or complete Fast and Long Menus using the instructions found in the Box above. Engage in several of these Distractions over the next couple of days and add them to your repertoire of Comfort Skills.

4. **Notice Positive Change.** In the days between now and the next Training Day, notice any large or small positive changes that enter your life and write them down. Ask yourself each day:

   **"What happened today, large or small,
   that I want to see more of in my life?"**

Flare Planning
Third Training Day – Week 6

The Skill Review

(A)
Re-Focusing Skills

For 20 minutes, practice Re-Focusing Skills #'s 1-5 or 7-8 found listed on page 338.

(B)
"I Want to See More of…"

Consult Journal or digital file, or review last several day, answer these questions:
- "What happened since the last Training Day, large or small, that I want to see more of in my life?"
- "What caused these things to happen?"

Today's Pain Problem
Pain Problem #7 – Underprepared for Pain Flares

Skills of the Day

Pain Flares – An Introduction
A **"Pain Flare"** *is an intense, and sometimes sudden, increase in your physical discomfort.* If you're unprepared for a pain flare, you're likely to feel helpless and you might panic. These reactions may cause you even more hurt and upset. Overall, you may feel unprepared to handle chronic pain and Misery, and this reinforces the false idea that you have no control over your life. However, you can take charge of the pain with a flare plan.

Fire Drills and Flare Plans
Remember when you were a kid in elementary school and the fire bell rang? Your teacher would quickly line you up and firmly instruct you to exit the classroom and walk to a safe place. When you were a kid in elementary school you were probably excited to get out of class for a while. Fire drills are a normal part of most educational institutions and they help children to reduce their anxiety when they're faced with an emergency situation. Escape plans and drills are also helpful for adults by preparing them to handle a fire or natural disasters such as earthquakes and hurricanes.

A pain flare is another kind of emergency situation. All of you know that the daily pain level you live with is bad enough without pain flares. As suggested above, when pain intensifies, it can drive you into a state of panic and emotional distress. Just as you follow an escape plan in the case of fire, you can follow another plan that helps you to reduce or at least better ride out a pain flare. It's very empowering because when the discomfort suddenly elevates, you won't need to think up any solutions on the spot – you just follow your Plan. As you do this, you'll return yourself to some level of Comfort, and diminish some of the pain and distress brought on by these temporary attacks.

STORY BOX #10 –
Carolyn's "Comfort Box"

Carolyn is a retired bank officer who came to see me a number of years ago. She is suffers from chronic low back pain and depression and, in the past, when a flare came along, she'd writhe in a tortured bed of pain and misery for at least two excruciating days. The increased pain intensity often pushed past the effect of her medication, which offered little relief. After some months attending my ongoing Comfort Circle support group, Carolyn carried a very large boot box in to a session. As she opened it up, she said,

"My Flare Plan is a "Comfort Box" that I can hold in my hands. It sits by my bed-stand and I only open it when the pain flares up. It has many of the things I enjoy - special CD's and DVD's, a Bible, chocolates, books, a list of people to send letters and emails to, a list of people to call for casual conversations, and a list of things I can look up on the Internet. As I rest up from the flare, I use these things to distract me from the pain and, usually, I feel more relaxed and in control."

Everyone in the group thought that the Comfort Box was a great idea and some made their own. Carolyn continues to use and benefit from her Box.

(A)
"Flare Planning in Sets of Three"

Just as there are many ways to set a goal, there are many formats you can use to create your own Flare Plan. Although these run the gamut from very basic to very comprehensive, I lean more toward the simple and straightforward. The Plan format below includes a combination of the Comfort Skills as well as practices you've developed yourself. After the next story, I'll detail options to creating a Pain Flare Plan in a Skill Box.

MOVING SKILL BOX #7 –
"Flare Planning in Sets of Three"

Step One - List Your Skills. Recall what practices you've done in the past that brought you some relief. Write them down in a journal or a digital file.

Step Two - Add New Comfort Skills to the List. Next, look over the Comfort Skills found in this book, and choose those that have been effective for you (see Chapter Three). Add them to your list.

Step Three - Organize the Top Nine into Sets of Three. Look over your list and choose nine of the most helpful Skills and personal resources. Follow this format:

A) Using your journal or a digital file, list these nine into sets of three, with the most useful sets towards the top.

B) Choose another nine and organize them the same way. Repeat this again and again until you have a collection of several "Sets of Three."

C) Transfer this Flare Plan to something you can carry with you (i.e., a 3x5 card, small calendar, or a smart phone).

D) (If you're not sure what Comfort Skills to use, choose from my sample Pain Flare Plan below.)

Step Four – Rehearse the Plan. Choose a time when you're not in a pain flare and rehearse your Plan in your mind. Imagine that the pain is flaring up and mentally experience yourself using each of the Skills in Sets of Three (IE, Imagine you are watching something funny on your I-Pad or TV).

Final Step –Use it for a Real Pain Flare. When you notice the First Sign of an impending flare, or if you've already begun to flare, pull out your list and begin to practice the Skills in the first Set of Three. After thirty minutes, if you're not comfortable enough, practice another Set of Three or repeat some on the first Set. Use as many Skills as you wish.

Remember

▪ Keep your Flare Plan handy, where you can get to it. After a while, you may have memorized parts of it and you won't need to look at it as often.

▪ *Replace desperate searching for pain relief with calm curiosity.* As you practice, notice what happens, allow the Comfort to come in its own time.

EXAMPLE BOX
"SETS OF THREE FLARE PLAN"

SITUATION *– You are washing the dishes and you feel a very intense and sharp ache in your shoulder. You recall that this usually warns you that a flare is on the way (a First Sign). Since you know that a full blown pain flare might be coming, you decide to take out your Flare Plan and practice the "Sets of Three" until you feel more at ease.*

The Flare Plan

Set Number One
   1) ***"Pay as You Go"*** - You take a break from the dishes and rest
   2) ***"Breath Count"*** – You sit in a comfortable seat and practice for 15 minutes
   3) ***"Laughing"*** – You watch a comedy DVD for at least 30 minutes

Set Number Two
   1) ***"Doing Fun"*** – You take a hot bath
   2) After your bath, you do some of your gentle stretches for 15 minutes
   3) ***"The Head Trip"*** – You practice for at least 15 minutes (perhaps imagining that you are on a beautiful island sunning yourself on the beach)

Set Number Three
   1) You call someone you'd love to talk with
   2) ***Positive Distraction – "The Fast Menu"*** – You surf the Internet for 30 minutes, or walk, bike, or drive to a pretty place, park somewhere and "people-watch"
   3) ***"Mantra/Breath Meditation"*** – For 20 minutes, you practice pairing a word (i.e., "calm") to your breath. Sound it out quietly in your mind with each exhale

(B)
"Two Bottles of Comfort" –

When faced with a flare up, most people in pain reach for their medicine bottles to help ease the pain. I'd like to "prescribe" a couple of different bottles for you thaqt you can use when the pain rises fast and hard: The Skill Bottle and the Flare Bottle. The Skill Bottle serves as a useful memory device that helps you recall what you can do to increase your Comfort level during an overwhelming pain flare. The Flare Bottle shows you how to carefully use your break-through-pain medications (i.e., Norco, Flexeril). (This Skill based on the perspective of a pain pharmacist colleague.)

MOVING SKILL BOX #8 –
"Two Bottles of Comfort"

The Skill Bottle

Step One -- Make a "Skill Bottle." Take a big, empty pill or vitamin bottle, tape a large, blank label around it, and write "Skill Bottle" on the top. Below the title, list at least ten to twenty Comfort Skills that offer you some relief. (Look through the Skills in "Appendix A" and also use your own resources.)

Step Two – "Candy Pills." Fill the bottle with your favorite little candies (i.e., chocolate-covered-raisins, M & M's, Pez candy).

Step Three – Go for the Skill Bottle. Each time you notice a First Sign of increasing pain or stress, stop what you're doing, grab your Skill Bottle, pull out a candy, and while you are eating it, choose one the Skills listed on the label and practice it (i.e., Meditation or watching a comedy). If you want more comfort, eat another candy and do another Skill (or repeat the first one).

Remember
- *SWEETS WARNING*. You might get tempted to eat a lot of candy. In order to prevent that, spend at least 20-to-30-minutes doing each Skill before you eat another piece of candy. Remember, one piece, one Skill.
- *Keep It Handy*. Keep your Skill Bottle with your medication and each time you take a pill, take a candy and use a Skill from that Bottle. You can also carry it with you wherever you go.

The Flare Bottle

The Flare Bottle comes in handy when the hurt rises and you've already used up you daily dose (for Short-Acting medications only). It puts you in control of your situation without creating any conflict with your doctors or putting you in danger of overdose or running out.

Step One – Make a "Flare Bottle." Take a big, empty pill or vitamin bottle, tape a large, blank label around it, and write "Flare Bottle" on the top. Below the title, write the name and dose of the pills it will contain (i.e., Norco, 325mg)

Step Two – Fill it on Good Days. On the days that you can go without using all of your Short-Acting medication, put the remaining pills in the Flare Bottle (i.e., If you only use three of your four daily Norco, put the extra one in the Flare Bottle.

Step Three – Use it on Bad Days. On high pain days when you've used your entire daily dose from your regular bottle and you are still hurting, you can take an extra pill or two from the Flare Bottle. For example, if your prescription is for one Norco every six hours (for a total of four a day), and the pain is still high after using all of your meds, you can take an extra pill from your Flare Bottle. Make sure to combine that with some Comfort Skills to add to your relief.

In other words→ "You can use a little more medication on some days as long as you use less on other days." In this way, you prevent yourself from running out.

Remember
- ***Talk with your doctor before you make and use a Flare Bottle.***
- WARNING - The type of medication should not be one that your physician says you need every day, such as long-acting Opiates (i.e., Morphine, Methadone, Suboxone). Only make a Flare Bottle for Short-Acting, break-through Opiates such as Norco or Percocet.
- Recall that even a safe dose of medication by itself will never give you enough relief. When you combine pills with Comfort Skills you'll increase your Comfort level beyond the medication effect.

The Last Practice
Re-Focusing Skills

For 20 minutes, practice a Re-Focusing Skill (see #'s 1-5 and 7-8 on page 338).

HOMEWORK BOX
THIRD TRAINING DAY – WEEK 6

1. **Practice Re-Focusing Skills.** Practice Re-Focusing Skills #'s 1-5 or 7-8 on page 338 for at least 20 minutes each day.

2. **Create Social Connections.** Continue to take steps towards spending social time with good people. If you already do this, do a little more (see pages 260-263).

3. **Make a Flare Plan.** Over the next few weeks, set up a Flare Plan as instructed above. Use it when you have a flare.

4. **Notice Positive Change.** In the days between now and the next Training Day, notice any large or small positive changes that enter your life and write them down. Ask yourself each day:

    "What happened today, large or small,
    that I want to see more of in my life?"

Week Seven – Dealing with Annoying People & Hypnosis
Eight Week Basic Training

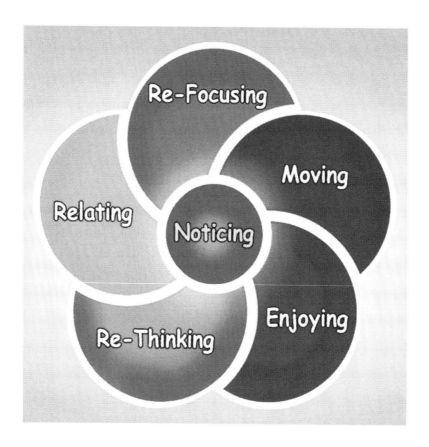

Pain Problems and Comfort Skill Solutions
Included in Week Seven

Pain Problems
- *"Attention Hijacked by Pain and Stress"*
- *"Sadness, Worry, & Other Miserable Feelings"*
- *"Hypersensitive Nervous System"*
- *"Distressed by Annoying People"*

Comfort Skill Solutions
- Direct Ways to Say No to Annoying People
- Indirect Ways to Say No to Annoying People
- "Self-Hypnosis – Three Inductions"

CONTENTS - WEEK SEVEN

Dealing with Annoying People Directly
First Training Day

1. The Skill Review
    - A) Re-Focusing Skill
    - B) *"I Want to See More of…"*
2. Today's Pain Problem
    - ▪ *"Pain Problem #6 - Distressed by Annoying People"*
3. Learn/About #21 - Annoying People
4. Learn/About #22 - Harmful Habits, Toxic Talk, and Saying "No!"
5. Skills of the Day
    - A) *"The C.A.L.M - Nice Guy Approach"*
    - B) *"The C.U.T. - Tough Guy Approach"*
6. The Last Practice
    - A) Re-Focusing Skill
7. Homework Box

Dealing with Annoying People Indirectly
Second Training Day

1. The Skill Review
    - A) Re-Focusing Skill
    - B) *"I Want to See More of…"*
2. Today's Pain Problem
    - ▪ *"Pain Problem #6 - Distressed by Annoying People"*
3. Skills of the Day
    - A) *"One Down Duck Down"*
    - B) *"Disarm Them in the Fog"*
    - C) *"Distracted Listening"*
4. The Last Practice
    - A) Re-Focusing Skill
5. Homework Box

Self-Hypnosis and Comfort
Third Training Day

1. The Skill Review
   A) Re-Focusing Skill
   B) *"I Want to See More of..."*
2. Today's Pain Problems
   ▪ *Pain Problem #2 - Attention is Hijacked by Pain and Stress*
   ▪ *Pain Problem #4 - Sadness Worry, and Other Miserable Feelings*
   ▪ *Pain Problem #9 - Hypersensitive Nervous System*
3. Learn/About #23 - Self-Hypnosis and Comfort
4. Skill of the Day (and Last Practice)
   A) *"Self-Hypnosis – Three Inductions"*
5. Homework Box

Dealing with Annoying People Directly
First Training Day – Week Seven

The Skill Review

(A)
Re-Focusing Skill

For 20 minutes, practice any Re-Focusing Skill (see #'s 1-5 and 7-8 on page 338).

(B)
"I Want to See More of..."

Consult your Journal or review the last several days and answer the two questions below.

- **"What happened since the last Training Day, large or small, that I want to see more of in my life?"**
- **"What caused these things to happen?"**

Today's Pain Problem
Pain Problem #6 – Distressed by Annoying People

Learn/About #21 – Annoying People

Most of us have known people who annoy us. According to the dictionary, the word "annoy" means to "disturb, harass, and irritate." **Annoying People** *are individuals you know, and may love, whose behavior and words make you feel uncomfortable and upset.* They are usually people who are close to you, like spouses, kids, family, friends, or neighbors. Others may include doctors, co-workers, or supervisors. Consider two types:

1. **Annoying People**. These folks may bother you occasionally (i.e., at bedtime), or regarding particular issues (i.e., finances, pain medication). Most of the time, you get along fairly well. Some of them annoy you from a place of good intention (i.e., one husband who wouldn't let his wife do anything around the house in order to protect her from pain). Whether they disturb you a little or a lot, the annoyance is limited.

2. **Seriously Annoying People.** These guys harass you most of the time. They often unknowingly push you into a full blown argument, rage, depression, panic attack, or pain flare. They might also irritate you on purpose. Some have a long history of annoying you, while others only began to treat you badly since chronic pain came into your life. Overall, you share very few happy or comfortable moments together.

The Skills in the Workbook will help with both types. However, when it comes to Seriously Annoying People, you may have to make long-term changes in order to find some happiness. No matter the type, Annoying People are annoying! Examples include:

- A spouse who talks down to you
- A mother or father who frequently criticizes your choices
- A doctor who sarcastically expresses disbelief that the pain is real
- A child or teenager who never does house chores and then hits you with an argument when you ask him or her to do something

Regardless how long they've bothered you, each time they do it your nervous system may become over-stimulated, your muscles tighten, and your mood sinks down. All of these effects lead to more stress, upset, and pain.

Reasoning with the Unreasonable

Annoying People will speak or act unreasonably towards you. When they engage in this, they may like a two-year-old who can use a large vocabulary to insult you. When you try to reason with them as a mature adult, they'll answer you like a petulant child, ignoring your good intentions and attacking you for your efforts. Or, they may talk down to you as if you were a child. If you continue to try negotiating with them, you'll make *one of the biggest mistakes you can make with these people: Attempting to reason with them when they are unreasonable.* When you make this mistake, you'll find yourself stuck in a harmful pattern that repeats itself again and again like a bad TV re-run – you may feel like you are hitting your head against the wall.

The Painful Relationship Pattern

The pattern of your interaction may go something like this:
- ➢ The Annoying Person says something hurtful
- ➢ Then you try to nicely talk with them about it
- ➢ Next, they answer you with more insults, manipulations, and/or emotional outbursts
- ➢ You again try to respond reasonably to them and the cycle starts over again

For example, one woman with a terrible back condition was pressured by her boyfriend to cook dinner for him every night (without his help). She tried to reasonably talk him out of it for 30 minutes to no avail. He kept nagging her and this filled her with feelings of guilt. Here, a reasonable person (the woman) tried to have a sincere conversation with someone who is unreasonable (the boyfriend). In the end, she felt miserable and gave in to his demands. You can guess what happened – each night after dinner, she suffered a severe pain flare.

What Does an Annoying Person Want? Some of these may seem familiar to you:

- ▪ **Annoying people want to get their way**. For example, they'll manipulate you to feel guilty in order to get you to do something they want. Usually, it's something that either upsets you or increases your pain level (i.e., hiking five miles), or, they may burden you with too many tasks and then refuse to help (i.e., clean the entire house).
- ▪ **Annoying people crave your attention**. This is big. It's highly valued by young people and adults alike. The more attention you give them while they are annoying you, the nastier they'll get and the longer they will bother you.
- ▪ **Annoying people want to invalidate you by arguing that they are right and you are wrong**. Like most people, you hold valid beliefs and take actions that are meaningful to you. Annoying people love to invalidate your beliefs and actions by demanding that their way of seeing things is right and yours is not.

When they achieve any or all of these goals, you'll most likely end up feeling angry, upset, or defeated. Again, you may also experience more pain.

Like the Person, Hate the Behavior

Let me make something very clear – <u>Annoying People are still people</u>. The above descriptions are intended to denigrate the people who make themselves annoying. Annoying

People may irritate you all (or even most) of the time, nor are they all fully aware about what they are doing. Many of them are fine people with whom you usually have good interactions. However, sometimes they have a tendency to talk to you in a hurtful manner. In the end, it is very important that you like the person (if possible) and hate their bad behavior. (This doesn't necessarily apply to "Seriously Annoying People.")

Learn/About #22 – Toxic Talk, Harmful Habits, Allies, and Saying "No!"

You may respond to an Annoying Person in ways that don't serve you well. Described below are three "Harmful Habits" that some of you engage in. As you probably know, the more you do them, the more they kill your Comfort. These include: 1) "Taking in Toxic Talk," 2) "Raging, Arguing, and Fighting," and 3) "Doing for Everyone but Yourself." (For a complete, annotated list of the twelve Harmful Habits, see Appendix B.)

"Taking in Toxic-Talk" - Harmful Habit #3 [90]

"Toxic Talk" *is the kind of message you receive from people who criticize, manipulate, threaten, guilt trip, and generally bad mouth you. Often, these words cause you to feel very uncomfortable.* When you "give in" and allow yourself to listen to their negative words you'll end up feeling upset. What's worse, as I've suggested in this training, when you feel emotionally distressed your nervous system becomes more sensitive to pain. When you spend too much time listening to the Annoying Person's poisonous words, you unintentionally allow them to put their Negative Thoughts into your head – and that hurts your body!

Toxic-Talk is Poisonous

That's right. It can hurt you even more than the pain because it poisons your body. How does that happen? It's no secret that Annoying People (and especially Seriously Annoying People) will stress you out. If you allow yourself to listen to their disturbing words or yelling day after day, you'll experience high levels of chronic stress, and this causes your body to fill up with lots of stress hormones turning your body into a bowl of "Stress Hormone Soup." (Your body is already overly stressed by pain and other difficulties.) When that occurs, your health becomes compromised. If your stress level stays high on a regular basis, it can cause or worsen diseases like high blood pressure or diabetes.[91] Toxic Talk also increases your pain level and also causes emotional harm, like feelings of abandonment and guilt.

---

[90] Find an annotated list of twelve "Harmful Habits" in Appendix B.
[91] You may find the following useful sources of information on stress and stress-related diseases: Read "Why Zebras Don't Get Ulcers" by Robert Sapolsky; also see http://en.wikipedia.org/wiki/Stress-related_disorders

In order to avoid the stress, pain, and disease that come from the hurtful words of Annoying People, **you need to walk away from them!** The longer you listen, the more poison you'll take into your system. When you stop "Taking in Toxic Talk," you protect yourself from its painful consequences.

Three Kinds of Toxic Talk

Three kinds of "Toxic Talk" that irritate you and add to your physical discomfort are 1) Criticism, 2) Manipulation, and 3) Intimidation. Too often, the Annoying Person has unknowingly trained you to predictably respond to their hurtful words and attitudes. This often makes you feel powerless. In other words, they create a "Problem Pattern" that you may unknowingly fall into.

Criticism

Annoying People may try to hurt you and "put you in your place" with criticism. The main message of this kind of Toxic Talk is that nothing you say or do is right or good. Knowingly or unknowingly, their goal is to invalidate you. Perhaps you've heard some of the following critical statements.

1. "That's not medicine, it's dope, which is what a drug addict like you depends on!"
2. "What a mess! Can't you get your butt up long enough to clean this house!?"
3. "What happened to the husband I used to have!?"
4. "We know that the 'pain' is just something you made up in your mind. You're such a head-case!"

In addition to using hurtful words, the Annoying Person's voice-tone is often nasty, belittling, and leaves you feeling invalidated as a person. For example, the sound of their voice may be condescending (i.e., "I don't think you can handle that activity") or angry (i.e., "YOU NEVER DO ANYTHING RIGHT!!!").

The Problem Pattern. Annoying People often use criticism to put you on the defensive and make you vulnerable to arguments. This is because they use particular words that get you to defend yourself and that may lead into some pretty bad fights and trampled feelings. A typical pattern looks like this:

- The Annoying Person unreasonably criticizes you (i.e., "you're a drug addict!")
- You try to reason with them by explaining the truth (i.e., "I'm using my prescription according to my doctor's advice").
- They shoot down what you just said (i.e., "You shouldn't use any prescriptions, your doctor knows nothing!").
- You might answer them by either:

> Nicely reasoning more and more (i.e., "Oh, but you don't understand, the doctor said it was safe to use this medicine"), or
> Angrily blowing up into a loud argument (i.e., "DAMN YOU! I SAID THAT THE DOCTOR SAID IT WAS OKAY! YOU ARE SO STUPID!!")

Both of these options typically result in hurt feelings and a pain flare.

Manipulation

Those who use manipulation want to get their way with you. They might want control, money, or attention. If you give in to them, you may end up doing things that lead to pain flares (i.e., washing, drying, folding, and putting away all the laundry, or working on your backyard for five hours straight). Manipulators are very talented in using guilt to get what they want at your expense. Their usual sales pitch leaves you feeling used, frustrated, and more miserable. Manipulative lines may include the following:

1. (Said to the kids in front of you), "Hey, guys, your mom said she doesn't want to go. What do you think about that?!"
2. "I'll talk with your boss if you keep using the drugs that doctor gave you."
3. "Come on, Dad, you know I'll pay you back. Why are you always thinking of yourself?!"

The Problem Pattern. Like advertising executives who use TV commercials, Annoying People use manipulation because it works! However, instead of using sex or status to sell you a product, the manipulator attacks you with guilt in order to get their way. You may find yourself giving in to the person just to shut them up. In part, this is because the longer you allow them to "sell" you, the more guilt and distress you feel. Ironically, the worse you feel, the more likely you are to take in the guilt. The manipulator knows how to keep you listening until you give them what they want. For some of you, it may seem like the "pain" of guilt feels worse than the chronic pain itself! You may do what they want and end up overdoing your activity. When that happen and the flare comes, you may mentally slap your forehead and think, "I let them do it again!"

Intimidation

Intimidation means to "make you timid; fill you with fear." It's an act that threatens you with harm or domination. The nefarious individuals who do this are more than annoying – they may be dangerous. A small number of them may end up going beyond threats to physical abuse and assault. However, most will use their words, voice tone, and body language to repeatedly harass and threaten you. Do any of these lines sound familiar?

1. (An angry husband yells) "WOMAN! DID YOU HEAR WHAT I SAID, DO IT NOW, OR ELSE!"

2. (A supervisor barks) "YOU THINK YOU CAN GET OUT OF YOUR CHAIR WHENEVER YOU FEEL LIKE IT!? DO YOUR JOB OR YOU WILL LOSE IT!"

3. (A live-in 20-year-old daughter screams into her mother's face) "CLEAN THE DISHES YOURSELF, BITCH!!"

The Problem Pattern. This may sound similar to the previous two Problem Patterns. The intimidator makes a threat and you back down, placate, and give in. All the while, she or he gets lots of your fearful attention. However, unlike the manipulator, this person wants you to cower before them. Intimidators want to show off their "power," and when they do, you may feel small, frightened, vulnerable and, of course, a lot of pain. If you argue, it could lead to a fight, to material or emotional loss, and to more pain. Even without physical violence present, your brain will go into RED ALERT, warning you that you are in a dangerous situation. Often, it feels like you are "walking on eggshells" when you're around them, fearing that any moment they will pounce. This sets off your "fight or flight" stress response, increasing fear and pain.

"Raging, Arguing, and Fighting"
Harmful Habit #4

This is a very painful Comfort Killer. It's probably obvious to you that when you fight with someone, you're going to get emotionally or physically hurt – even if you "win" the argument. As we learned earlier, when you get angry & excited during an argument, your nervous system becomes more sensitive to the pain.

There is nothing more infuriating than when an Annoying Person pulls you into an argument. Many of the things they say and do will enrage you to the point that you'll raise your voice and get very angry. Although this might feel "good" in the moment, afterwards you'll probably get emotionally upset, physically tense, and experience more body aches. Also, your mind will be buzzing with instant replays of the fight, which stresses your nervous system and builds up even more bad feelings. The solution to this is obvious and not very easy to do at first – avoid the fight. As I discussed above, you can best do this by getting away from the Toxic Talk that "invites" you to argue. Even if you are in the middle of an argument, you can make a powerful "U-Turn" by walking away (See Skill Boxes below).

When it comes to this Harmful Habit, it is important that you remember this:
When You Argue, Even When You Win, You Lose

"Doing for Everyone but Yourself"
Harmful Habit #2

The title of this Harmful Habit says it all. Some of you habitually work against your own best interests by helping everyone in your life except you. In the end, you'll attract people who are very willing to suck the life out of you. This happens because you're always saying "yes" to their requests. Those who are already in your social world expect you to sacrifice your needs in order to fulfill theirs. The next story clearly shows you what this can look like.

STORY BOX #30 – Mona the Yes Girl

Most of the people in Mona's life loved her because she helped them whenever they asked (or demanded). For example, her physically healthy mother would call her day or night and get her to come over and do laundry or run an errand. None of Mona's other three siblings would do this – they expected her to take on the role as "Mom's servant." Mona would also snap to it each time her lazy, live-in boyfriend asked her for a "favor." For example, he usually expected her to drive to his ex-wife's house, pick up his two young daughters, bring them home, and take care of them during his "visitation time."

All of this giving brought her a lot of misery. Aside from the fact that she rarely did things that she wanted, Mona would end up overdoing her activity and getting a pain flare. Her left leg would quiver with a searing pain from an injury she sustained in her twenties. The stress of "having no life" depressed her and ate her up on the inside. However, she felt compelled to do somebody else's bidding because if she didn't, Guilt would hound her or her mother or boyfriend would play their own "guilt soundtrack" and nag her until she gave in.

For example, once she had a severe flare in her leg and she told her boyfriend, "I don't think that I can pick up the girls today." He manipulated her by saying, "Mona, I'm in the middle of this project and I can't get away. You don't want the girls to miss their visit, do you?" Mona then sadly responded, "Oh, okay. Yes, I'll get them." The shame that she felt caused her to cave in and drive thirty painful minutes to his ex-wife's house to get the kids. Later that day, she found herself in bed writhing in a major pain flare.

As in so many other situations, Mona had a difficult time saying the word that would have saved her from this flare. This word, when hurled at the Manipulators in her life, would also protect her and give her time to herself.

And yes → that word is "No!" Later, Mona benefitted by saying it.

Pain's Ally vs Your Ally

Before learning the Skills that help you disarm Annoying People, you'll find it useful to think about the idea of allies. An **"Ally"** *is someone (or even a skill or action) that helps you stand up to an opponent or problem*. Your Ally works with you against chronic pain and his Cronies (i.e., Depression). Below is a true story that illustrates this.

STORY BOX #31 - A Great Guy

Doug was Joanie's boyfriend and he loved her a lot. He showed just how much he cared for her on the day of her auto collision. It wasn't much of a fender bender – someone hit her car from behind going about five miles-per-hour. At worst, it would have been a bit of a sore neck for a couple of months. The problem was, Joanie already had a damaged neck from a hit-and-run accident that she survived five years before. As you might imagine, her pain level went through the roof after this second, "minor" accident. Doug rushed to the hospital immediately and did not leave her side. Because they couldn't get a hold of her regular doctor, the emergency room staff wouldn't give Joanie any additional pain medication because they said that "she had a lot of pills already." They also said that her injuries "did not warrant it." Doug acted as her advocate, speaking to successive hospital staff until he was able to appeal to the physician in charge to give Joanie enough extra pain pills to last until her doctor returned.

Doug's support did not end there. First, over the next few weeks, he took on some of Joanie's house tasks. He also reminded her to practice her Comfort Skills. (She had earlier coached him on how he could remind her to take care of herself when she became too overwhelmed by pain and stress.) From time to time, he'd quietly look into her eyes when she was distressed and say the words she taught him: "It's time for a break now, okay?" This signaled her to stop what she was doing and either practice twenty minutes of Meditation or do something pleasurable, like hold her little dog in her lap and brush his hair. Finally, Doug buffered her from family and friends who tried to pressure her to take on more activities than she could comfortably do. For a good while, she left to Doug the task of talking with them. This freed her from hearing their Toxic alk.

All of Doug's help made it possible for Joanie to recover from this major pain flare within a month. A great deal of this quick recovery was due to how well Doug acted as her Ally against pain and distress.

Say "No!" to Annoying People

The Relating Skill provided in this section can help you to:
- ❖ Say "No!" to the unreasonable demands of Annoying People
- ❖ Say "No!" to their manipulation and guilt-tripping
- ❖ Say "No!" to their criticisms and threats

A friend of mine once told me that "No!" is the new "Yes." See how below.

STORY BOX #8 – Monique Says "No!"

Despite the searing pain that 45-year-old Monique felt in her left foot, she was still able to work part-time as a receptionist in a large medical office. She was a very good worker and took on more than just receptionist duties. This was because, in order to save money on additional staff, her office manager expected her to take on more work than she was required. She was afraid to refuse him.

Several times a week, she'd lift and carry heavy boxes and stack forms on high shelves, causing her a lot of pain. A number of times when one of her supervisor's favorite employees gave him a last-minute request for time off, he'd ask/demand Monique to come into work on her day off. Each time he did this, she'd give in with little complaint. However, later on, her stress level intensified and this resulted in a terrible pain flare. On top of that, when she tried to call in sick after one of these flares, her supervisor would give her a hard time on the phone and pressure her to come in that day. Since she was afraid she'd lose her job, Monique would go to work in a flare and squirm all day in a chair of pain.

After she told us this sad story in the Comfort Workshop, the group members gave her a great deal of support to stand up for her rights. They also told her that she was his best, and most dependable, worker, one who is very difficult to replace. This encouraged her to deal with her manager differently.

Monique didn't have to wait long to test this out because at the end of the next day, her boss told her he needed her to stay "a little longer." Amazingly…she said, "No!" At first, he was taken aback. Then, he launched into a long, rambling speech about her obligations to their department. She knew there was no reasoning with him and so she cut him off, saying, "Sorry, Ralph, I can't do that anymore. I'm going home, see you tomorrow." She turned around and walked out, leaving him with his jaw hanging down to the floor. She did the same thing on a couple of other occasions and eventually he stopped asking. After that, her job became a much more comfortable place to work.

Two Ways to Say "No!" – Direct and Indirect Limit Setting

Two Skill-Sets empower you to firmly and effectively say "No!" to Toxic Talk.

1. The **Direct Limit Skill-Set** provides you with Skills that help you meet the challenges these people put before you. It arms those of you who are prepared to directly confront and set limits on the annoying behavior. The Skill provided below is Direct Limit Setting.

2. The **Indirect Limit Skill-Set** does this in a powerfully round-about fashion. It's for those of you who find it too difficult to directly confront the offending individual. It's made up of subtle tactics that disarm the offending person in a way that is not obvious to them. I offer three of these Skills in the Second Training Day of this Week (see page 298).

WARNING!!! – Be Cautious Around Annoying People in Power

Some Annoying People have the power to harm you financially, emotionally, or physically (i.e., your boss at work, a controlling husband who manages the bank account). If you are in a vulnerable position, you should seek the advice of a counselor, a therapist, a lawyer, or the police before confronting this type of Annoying Person. Reserve the use of these Skills for people who will not seriously harm you.

STORY BOX #32 – Leilani "Meditates"

Leilani is a 29-year-old woman who suffered from terrible migraine headaches and neck pain. Although her husband was wonderful most of the time, there were times (at least once a week) when he would become cranky and very irritating. This usually pulled Leilani into a loud, angry argument, which caused a headache.

In the middle of one yelling match, she remembered that she didn't want another argument or headache, and she also recalled that Negative Thoughts were "nothing" and had no power over her unless she followed them. Using this knowledge and combining it with a Re-Focusing Skill, Leilani put her hand out like she was stopping traffic and said to her husband, "You're just a thought! I'm going to meditate now. I'll talk to you later."

Then, she quickly and calmly turned around, walked into a quiet room, sat down comfortably, and meditated for 20 minutes. Interestingly, she became aware that her husband quietly came in and out of the room a couple of times. She later found out that he was checking on her to make sure that she was okay. In the end, the argument was forgotten and they had a peaceful evening. Headache was nowhere to be seen.

Skills of the Day

Direct Limit-Setting –
The "C.A.L.M." and "C.U.T." Approaches

There is a simple difference between these two techniques:

- The **"C.A.L.M. – Nice Guy Approach"** is very effective with Annoying People who will change their behavior when you ask them to stop bothering you.

- The **"C.U.T." – Tough Guy Approach"** was designed for those individuals who will test you to see if you really want to be treated decently. Even though you have asked them in the past to treat you with respect, they will continue to annoy you and even criticize you for asking them to stop their Toxic Talk. The "Tough Guy Approach" is more forceful and empowers you to leave the Annoying Person's Toxic Talk far behind!

(A)
"The C.A.L.M. Nice Guy Approach"

This Skill is very effective with people who are willing to change their behavior when you ask them to stop abusing you. These folks need a little reminder about what you'll do if they don't stop their Toxic Talk. If you're prepared to firmly (and effectively) stand up to an Annoying Person and their bad words and behavior, then this is the right Skill for you.

RELATING SKILL BOX #3 - "The C.A.L.M. Nice Guy Approach"

Step One – Ask Yourself the "Personal 1-2-3." Annoying kids and adults confront you with their "1-2-3" → 1) I want, 2) what I want, 3) when I want it. A powerful way to counter this is with your own 1-2-3. When someone is annoying you, ask yourself the following:

- *One – "What Do I Want?"* This is critical and we often forget to ask ourselves this. Example Answers – "I want him to stop criticizing me," or, "I want her to stop asking me how I feel."
- *Two – "When Do I Want it to Happen?"* What are your time needs? Right now? In an hour? When you spell this out for yourself you leave no wiggle room for the Annoying Person to change the time.
- *Three – "What Will I Do if I Don't Get It?"* You can create and impose <u>consequences</u> on the offending person if they don't comply with your request. Examples:
  - ➢ Remove your attention by walking away
  - ➢ Briefly take away a misbehaving child's privileges (i.e., I-Pad)

Step Two – Use the C.A.L.M. Nice Guy Approach. Carry out your own "Personal 1-2-3."

Cut Off. Interrupt the person talking. If you don't stop the Toxic Talk, it will go on and on. Although this may feel like an impolite interruption, it's not. Useful Cut-Off lines include:

- "Excuse me."
- "Let's stop for a moment."
- "Wait! I have to tell you something."

You can even hold your hand up as if you are stopping traffic.

Alert & Ask. Briefly **Alert** them by saying that their words are irritating, frustrating, or hurtful. Then, **Ask** them in a sentence or two what you clearly want from them. For example:

- "You're words are upsetting me right now" (<u>Alert</u>), and
- "I want you to stop talking to me that way right now!" (<u>Ask</u>)

Limit. Add to the end of your request a warning that if you don't get what you're asking for, you may have to do something they won't like – usually removing your attention from them by walking away. You can phrase the Limit using an **"If - Then Statement,"** said either in the negative or positive:

- <u>*Negative Example*</u> - "**If** you don't stop criticizing me, **Then** I'm going out for a while by myself."
- <u>*Positive Example*</u> - "**If** you stop criticizing me, **Then** we can talk."

Move On to Something Good. If the person doesn't stop their Toxic Talk or upsetting behavior, <u>the discussion is **OVER**</u>. No more talking or reasoning with them. Tell them that you'll see them later and then "Move On" by walking away for a while. How do you do this? – <u>Turn around and follow your feet!</u> But that is not all – in order to clean out any bad feelings caused by their Toxic Talk, its best to do something enjoyable. The more upset you are, the bigger the pleasure you deserve. You can return to the person later, when they've either apologized or begun to speak to you with more respect and care.

"Fly-Fishing" Alert!!

If you have to walk away, the Annoying Person may try to pull you back into the argument with lines like "There you go, leaving again!" or "What kind of wife/husband are you!?" Don't fall for this "fly fishing" – just follow your feet out of the room and "Move on to Something Good."

STORY BOX #9 –
Cindy Stays C.A.L.M.

Cindy's father was always nagging her about her work habits. Since she survived a car accident three years ago, Cindy changed her way of carrying out her tasks. She worked for a publishing company as an editor and her boss allowed her to do book editing assignments in her home and at her own pace. She'd work at her home computer station and take a lot of breaks. This allowed her to feel more Comfort over the constant pain she felt in her back.

Unfortunately, this wasn't good enough for her father, a "self-made-man" who advanced in his company to become a vice-president for sales. Again and again, on the phone or face-to-face, he'd bring up how she "should be more active" and "go to work like everybody else." Most times, Cindy came away from his nagging sessions exhausted and depressed. Sometimes, she yelled back at him and this made things worse.

When Cindy learned about the C.A.L.M. Skill, she decided to use it on her father to stop his Toxic Talk. One Monday, he came to her house for a visit and found her taking a break on her recliner. Seeing this, he began to criticize her for being "lazy." Cindy "Saw it Coming," continued sitting comfortably in her chair, and did the following:

- *Cut Off.* Holding up her hand, she said, "Dad, wait a minute."
- *Alert & Ask.* "When you criticize me like that, I feel very bad and it does not help me to work or feel comfortable. I'd like you to stop talking about how I work and change the subject to something more positive."
- *Limit.* "If you can do that, then I want you to stay and we can have a nice visit. But, if you feel that you have to keep criticizing me and telling me what to do, then let's stop talking now and I'll see you later."
- *Move on to Something Good.* Sadly, her father could not respect her request, so she told him to leave. Even though she felt relief from his nagging, she felt bad about the interaction they had. To return herself to a happier state, she decided to accept that she'd feel bad for a while. While she waited for the mood to pass, she took a nice walk and then watched a funny video.

Later, Cindy told me that this Skill worked like a charm and it prevented her father and Guilt from bringing her down. What was even better - as she continued to meet her dad's guilt tripping with this Relating Skill, he annoyed her less and less.

(B)
"The C.U.T. -- Tough Guy Approach"

Use this option with people who appear to have no intention of changing their behavior, even after you've given them a chance in the past to stop annoying you.

RELATING SKILL BOX #4-
"The C.U.T. -- Tough Guy Approach"

Step One – Ask Yourself the Personal "1-2-3." Annoying kids and adults confront you with a "1-2-3" - 1) I want, 2) what I want, 3) when I want it. A powerful way to counter this is with your own 1-2-3:

- *One – "What Do I Want?"* We often forget to ask ourselves this question. Example answer – "I want him to stop criticizing me."
- *Two – "When Do I Want it to Happen?"* What are your time needs? Right now? In an hour? When you spell this out for yourself you leave no wiggle room for the Annoying Person to change the time.
- *Three – "What Will I Do if I Don't Get It?"* You can create and impose <u>consequences</u> on the offending person if they don't comply with your request. Examples:
- Remove your attention by walking away
- Briefly take away a misbehaving child's privileges (i.e., iPod)

Step Two - C.U.T. Them Off at the Knees! No need to reason with them anymore. Free yourself from their abuse by using the C.U.T. Skill.

Cut Off. If you don't interrupt the Toxic Talk they will go on and on or say things to get you to argue or endlessly defend yourself. It's up to you to stop their ranting. Although this may feel like an impolite interruption, it's not. Useful Cut-Off lines include:

➢ "Excuse me,"
➢ "Let's stop for a moment,"
➢ "Wait! I have to tell you something."

You can also hold your hand up like you are stopping traffic.

U –Turn. No matter where you are in your discussion with them, make a "U-turn" by getting ready to remove yourself from their presence. Ignore any thoughts that tell you that it's not okay to leave in the middle of a discussion – get ready to go. Before you turn around, it's best to say a brief exit-line before you turn your body around to walk away. Try one of these:

> ➤ Straight Exit-Line = "I've got to take a time out; see you later."
> ➤ Funny Exit-Line = "Oh my god! My pants are on fire. Gotta go!"

Take a Walk Towards Something Good. Ignore anything they say (short of an apology or a reasonable offer to talk). Turn around and follow your feet as they walk you away from the Annoying Person! Be aware that the person may try to pull you back by throwing lines at you like "There you go, leaving again!" Don't fall for this "fly fishing" – just keep going. As you walk away, move towards something that you enjoy. The more upset you are, the bigger the pleasure you deserve; you can draw from your "Fun Menu" (page 162). Later, if they sincerely apologize or speak to you with more respect and care, you can return to your usual relationship time with them.

The Last Practice
Re-Focusing Skill

For 20 minutes, practice a Re-Focusing Skill (see #'s 1-5 and 7-8 on page 338).

HOMEWORK BOX
FIRST TRAINING DAY – WEEK 7

1. **Practice a Re-Focusing Skill.** Select one of Re-Focusing Skills #'s 1-5 or 7-8 on page 338 and practice it for at least 20 minutes each day.

2. **Imagine Setting a Direct Limit.** Review the two Relating Skills above and imagine applying one to a difficult interaction you've had with an Annoying Person.

3. **Notice Positive Change.** In the days between now and the next Training Day, notice any large or small positive changes that enter your life and write them down. Ask yourself each day:

> "What happened today, large or small,
> that I want to see more of in my life?"

Dealing with Annoying People Indirectly
Second Training Day – Week Seven

The Skill Review

(A)
Re-Focusing Skill

For 20 minutes, practice a Re-Focusing Skill on page 338.

(B)
"I Want to See More of…"

Consult your Journal, or review the last several days and answer the two questions below.

- "What happened since the last Training Day, large or small, that I want to see more of in my life?"
- "What caused these things to happen?"

Today's Pain Problem
Pain Problem #6 – Distressed by Annoying People

Skills of the Day

The Indirect Way to Say "No!"

A number of you may have a hard time directly standing up to an annoying individual or group. The Indirect approach is useful if you've tried the Direct Approach and it didn't work as well as you hoped. It comprises several methods that can also stop the Toxic Talk and bad behavior aimed at you.

(A)
"One-Down Duck Down"

One unhelpful quality that Annoying People can bring out of us is the defensiveness. This Skill prevents them from pushing you into this ineffective behavior.

RELATING SKILL BOX #5 -
"One-Down Duck Down"

The Problem. When an Annoying Person assaults you with their poisonous words, it's as if they are verbally punching you in the face. They may raise your defensiveness and cause you to talk yourself into exhaustion or drag you into an angry fight. Others of you may decide to stand there and take it. All of these responses may create more pain and more emotional upset.

The "One-Down, Duck Down" Solution. A powerful way to avoid this situation and "disarm" their attacks is to take a *"One-Down"* position by seeming to agree with the aggressor's Toxic Talk. When you say this with an actor's voice of sincerity, it's as if you verbally *"Duck Down"* and the Annoying Person's negative words just fly over your head and miss you.

Walk Away. Once you've said your piece, follow your feet away from them and go do something fun.

Example Story

Sandra had a difficult time saying "No!" to her aunt, who would always boss her around and use guilt to manipulate her. Sandra had diabetes and one day her aunt baked a sweet cake and pressured her to eat this unhealthy snack. When she refused, her aunt told her that she was being a very selfish and disrespectful niece. Sandra "Ducked Down" by calmly saying, *"Oh, Auntie, I'm sorry but you are right. I am disrespectful and I'll probably never be a good enough niece."* As she walked away, she sincerely said to her aunt, *"This makes me very sad. Please excuse me. I have to go away now and be alone."* Sandra took herself out to the movies that day and had a good time.

(B)
"Disarm Them in the F.O.G"

This Relating Skill can empower you to take the punch out of the Annoying Person's Toxic Talk and move you away from it and towards something more positive and desirable.

RELATING SKILL BOX #6 -
"Disarm Them in the F.O.G"

F.O.G. The following three actions can free you from the unreasonable, irritating hold of an Annoying Person.

Fake It with No Blame. When they harangue you with Toxic Talk, "act as if" you're very sad, tired, or disoriented (see Hassi's Story below). Tell the person that you feel bad and don't know why; never blame them. If they accuse you of blaming them, deny it or apologize for "accidentally" blaming them. Continue to reassure them that you don't know why you feel bad. At the same time, keep acting clueless and helpless.

Offer Hidden Consequence with No Blame. Get ready to remove your attention and <u>Do Not</u> tell them what you're doing. Instead, pretend that you are in a "helpless state," and politely, apologetically excuse yourself, saying, *"I'm sorry, I'm just feeling too sad (...tired...ill) to talk now. I have to _____ (go lie down, take a walk, etc.) I'll talk with you later."* (Sometimes this works even if they know you're acting.)

Go. This Skill only works when you turn around and walk away. Do it a little slowly and don't stop no matter what "fishing lines" they throw at you to get you to come back. Stay "in character," acting like a depressed, tired, and/or confused person. Either go lie down to rest, take a walk, or do something enjoyable to take care of yourself. This enables you to get away from the Annoying Person and their Toxic Talk without directly confronting them. After you return, repeat the **F.O.G**. if they continue their Toxic Talk.

STORY BOX #33 – Hassi FOG's the Husband

Hassi was married to a very argumentative husband. Even though he was a nurse, he had little compassion for her. She suffered a great deal from the full-body pain of Fibromyalgia. This condition limited what tasks she could accomplish around the house. Although today she is no longer home-bound, she used to stay home most of the time. Her now ex-husband would come home every day from work and he'd either nag her about her use of medication or criticize her for being "lazy." In this way, he acted like a dedicated ally to Pain. His criticism would either depress her or pull her into a "knock down drag out" fight. As you might imagine, this caused her untold suffering and that made her miserable.

Hassi was a shy person who didn't feel that she could directly confront her husband about his hurtful speech. However, she liked the idea of using the F.O.G. Skill, so we co-created a plan during our weekly therapy session. The next week, soon after her husband returned from work, this is what happened:

- *Fake It* – He soon launched into a tirade of nagging, criticizing, and guilt-tripping. Hassi was ready for this and calmly listened to him while he spoke down to her. As planned, after a few minutes, she began to slowly lower her eyes to the floor and sighed four very deep sighs. Her husband sarcastically asked, "What is going on with that!"

- *Offer Hidden Consequence with No Blame* - She said, "I don't know; I just feel really low and tired. I think I better go lie down for a while. I'll talk to you later."

- *Go* - Hassi slowly turned around, walked to her room, lay down, and rested.

What her husband did not know was that <u>this was all an act</u>. He also didn't know what to do, so, he stopped talking and went to watch TV. She did this each time he tried to criticize or argue with her and, in time, he cut down on criticizing her after work. Even though her home became more peaceful, she soon realized that the relationship was not worth staying in, so one day, she moved on.

(C)
"Distracted Listening"

Often, when faced with a barrage of criticism or guilt tripping, we feel like closing out ears to the toxicity of the Annoying Person's nagging. This next Skill invites you to do this on purpose with the strategic goal of setting an indirect limit on their Toxic Talk.

RELATING SKILL BOX #7 -
"Distracted Listening"

Pretending. When someone is talking badly to you, you can intentionally and secretly pretend that you're listening to them, although you really aren't. You just stay silent and pretend that you are listening while they blather on and on.

Who is this Option For? This Skill is best practiced if:
- You don't feel that you can directly say "No!" to them
- You're very hesitant to walk away while the Annoying Person is verbally abusing you
- You're able to temporarily ignore or tolerate their Toxic Talk

Here's How to Do It. When the annoying individual hassles you, pretend that you're listening and avoid adding to the conversation or giving him or her any eye contact. (If they insist that you look into their eyes, look at their forehead.) As they talk, you can think about other things, such as what you plan to do that day, or replay an old movie in your head, or think about a good experience you had in the past.

- *If they don't notice that you're doing this, that's okay* - just wait until they're done, then walk away and do something you enjoy in order to clear out the negativity they just spewed all over you.
- *If they accuse you of not listening to them* - then apologize for "spacing out," and excuse yourself, saying, *"I'm probably too tired and distracted to listen now; I'll listen later."* Go lie down and rest, or do a pleasant activity.
- *Later, if you find yourself facing them again as they criticize you* - repeat this Skill. If they complain that "you never listen," pretend to be confused by saying something like, *"I don't know what's happening; I'm just not able to focus well lately. Let's try again sometime later."* Then, walk away.

The Last Practice
Re-Focusing Skills

For 20 minutes, practice a Re-Focusing Skills on page 338.

HOMEWORK BOX
SECOND TRAINING DAY – WEEK 7

1. **Practice a Re-Focusing Skill.** For 20 minutes, practice one of the Re-Focusing Skills on page 338 (#'s 1-5 or 7-8).

2. **Rehearse Setting an Indirect Limit in Your Imagination.** Review the three Indirect Skills above, and imagine applying them to a difficult interaction you've had with an Annoying Person. If you decide to imagine using the "Disarm them in the F.O.G.," perhaps you'll do what Hassi did in her situation (see Story Box above).

3. **Notice Positive Change.** In the days between now and the next Training Day, notice any large or small positive changes that enter your life and write them down. Ask yourself each day:

    **"What happened today, large or small,
    that I want to see more of in my life?"**

Self-Hypnosis and Comfort
Third Training Day – Week 7

The Skill Review

(A)
Re-Focusing Skills

For 20 minutes, practice a Re-Focusing Skill on page 338.

(B)
"I Want to See More of…"

Consult your Journal, or review the last several days and answer the two questions below.

- **"What happened since the last Training Day, large or small, that I want to see more of in my life?"**
- **"What caused these things to happen?"**

Today's Pain Problems

Pain Problem #2 – Attention Hijacked by Pain and Stress
Pain Problem #9 – "Hypersensitive Nervous System"
Pain Problem #4 – "Sadness, Worry, and Other Miserable Feelings"

Learn/About #23 – Self-Hypnosis & Comfort

Of all the Focusing Skills, this is by far the most powerful. More research than I can mention here has shown how Hypnosis increases your feelings of Comfort. Below, I will introduce you to three different techniques you can use. However, you will gain a lot by first learning a little about this Skill. The following pages will introduce you to some of the background of Hypnosis. If you wish to learn more than what is offered in this book, it's probably best to consult a reputable clinical hypnotist.[92]

---

[92] One source is ASCH.net.

Self-Hypnosis – A Brief Introduction

Okay, let's get this out of the way before we get started – here are some myths and facts about this Re-Focusing Skill:

Hypnosis is not:

- **Mind control** – however, you can learn how to use your mind to help your body
- **Only something that someone does to you** – even when a hypnotist guides you, you are ultimately in control of the process. In other words, "All Hypnosis is Self-Hypnosis"
- **Voodoo, magic, or some satanic ritual** – it won't "possess" you or cause you to do anything wrong or immoral

Hypnosis is:

- **A powerful Re-Focusing Skill** - It increases relaxation and puts you in charge of your attention
- **An effective tool that increases Comfort**
- **An established clinical treatment** - It was developed by healers, clinicians, and scientitsts over the last two centuries

Many studies carried out over the last century have demonstrated the efficacy of Hypnosis in relieving pain, calming anxiety, and soothing emotional upset.[93] The next story relates how, early on, Hypnosis was an effective remedy for surgical pain.

STORY BOX #32 – Dr. Esdaile's Treatment

Doctor James Esdaile empathized deeply with the surgical patients he treated in a British medical clinic established in India. It was the early 1840s and chemical anesthesia had not been invented yet. Fifty percent of these patients died under the surgeon's knife. This was due to the traumatic shock of extreme physical pain caused by amputations, tumor removals, and other procedures.

---

[93] "Essentials of Hypnosis" by Michael Yapko (This is an excellent introduction to Hypnosis by one of the most eminent psychologists and hypnotists in the United States).

Dr. Esdaile decided to do something about this problem and he started using a relatively new technique that put people to "sleep," numbed parts of their bodies, and calmed their spirits. It was called "Mesmerism," named after its Austrian inventor, Franz Anton Mesmer (today, we call it "Hypnosis"). Dr. Esdaile first used it in 1845 on a man who needed surgery on his genitals. You can just imagine how sensitive that would have been! However, after the man was hypnotized, he felt no sensitivity and no pain. This caused the surgery and recovery to go very well.

This encouraged Dr. Esdaile to regularly use this method on other patients and, over time, he found that Hypnosis helped them to have more comfortable recoveries. Most of the 3000 Hypnosis patients he operated on were fairly at ease during and after surgery. This included 300 people who underwent major surgery (i.e., amputation). He reported that the death rate from traumatic shock reduced from 50% to 5%! In 1848, because of these successes, Dr. Esdaile was provided an entire hospital dedicated to the use and study of Hypnosis as a treatment for medical patients. In 1891 the British Medical Association proclaimed: "As a therapeutic agent, hypnotism is frequently effective in relieving pain, procuring sleep and alleviating many functional ailments."

Unfortunately, most physicians did not practice this technique and it fell into complete disuse in the late 1840s after the discovery of ether and other chemical anesthetics. Today, Hypnosis is still used for surgical patients who do not respond well to chemical anesthesia. It's also practiced by some women going through child birth.

For over one hundred years, Hypnosis has been recognized as a legitimate treatment for pain.[94] If medical patients can learn how to control the pain caused by a surgeon's knife, do you think you can learn how to do the same with chronic pain? Below, I'll answer that question by giving you three Hypnosis Scripts that will train you in the use of hypnosis. It is not necessary for you to read the next section in order to practice.

If you want to start the training right now, skip to the "Skills of the Day" section (on page 311). However, if you want to learn a little more about Hypnosis, turn the page and continue reading.

---

[94] References include the following: a) www.uktraining.co.uk/james-esdaile.html, c) "Hidden Depths: The Story of Hypnosis," by Robin Waterfield

Hypnosis and the Brain

Contemporary studies over the last century discovered that the power of the mind over the nervous system and pain is very significant. MRI and PET scans reveal particular parts of the brain that are affected by Hypnosis.[95]

Hypnosis – What is it?

What exactly is Hypnosis? Here is the simple answer: we don't know. We do know that it's very effective in treating a diverse number of problems including Chronic Pain, discomfort from childbirth and other medical conditions, harmful eating and smoking habits, sleeplessness, test anxiety, warts and skin diseases, and depression and anxiety. However, even though we haven't discovered exactly what it is, it may be more important to understand what it can do for you.

Hypnotic Trance and Inductions?

Hypnosis has been described in a variety of ways. In order to clarify how it's used in this training program, it's important that you read these two definitions:

1. **Trance**. Some hypnotists describe the experience of Hypnosis as a "Trance." This is defined as a special state of mind characterized by deep relaxation, absorbed attention, high suggestibility, and enhanced imagination.[96] These are harnessed to help you make desired changes (i.e., alter the nervous system to reduce pain). I agree with those scientists and practitioners who have observed that Trance is actually a ***natural state*** we go in and out of on a regular basis (i.e., while watching a movie in a theater).[97]

2. **Inductions**. These are a set of instructions that you, or the hypnotist, use to guide you into a Trance. For example, when the hypnotist counts from ten down to one, then offers some ideas of comfort, and you allow yourself to close your eyes and follow those numbers and ideas, you're likely to move into a relaxed, hypnotic state.

Hypnosis – Adding a Third Re-Focusing Action

Recall in earlier chapters that I discussed two Actions that are common to most Re-Focusing Skills. When you do these, you begin to change your physiology and nervous system for the better. To review, the first two Actions are:

---

[95] See David Patterson, "Clinical Hypnosis for Pain Control," and Mark Jensen, "Hypnosis for Chronic Pain Management."

[96] See Michael Yapko, "Trancework: An introduction to the practice of clinical hypnosis."

[97] This "natural trance" was first observed by the great psychiatrist and innovator of hypnosis, Milton H. Erickson (see www.Erickson-Foundation.org).

- **Action One – "Let Go and Relax."** The first thing to do is relax your mind and body as best you can. Allow your muscles to soften and let thoughts, feelings, sounds, or other distractions come and go without dwelling on or fighting them. Just let them be there and take on a "laid back attitude." Do your best to chill out and take it easy. In this way, you'll release the distractions and prevent yourself from trying too hard to <u>make</u> something happen. When you notice that you are distracted by something, just let it go and return to focus. Allow the Comfort to come in its own time.

- **Action Two – "Focus on One Thing."** As you "Let Go and Relax," you also "Focus on One Thing" by aiming your attention, like a laser beam, at something pleasant or neutral. Keep your focus there. You might concentrate on your breath, on the sound of water, on a happy memory, or even on a good word repeated over and over in your mind, or focus on two things at once (i.e., breath & Mantra word).

When you put these two actions together, you can change your physiology and enhance your health and comfort. If you've been using any of the previously mentioned Re-Focusing Skills, you've already been practicing two-thirds of what you do in Self-Hypnosis. As you Let Go and Focus on the voice of the hypnotist, or on your "inner voice," you'll be able to do the following third Action:

- **Action Three – "Take in Ideas."** When you "Take in Ideas" from the hypnotist (or yourself), your Inner Mind will use them to help you develop positive experiences. What's great about this is that the only thing you need to do is allow it to happen. In other words, let useful words come in and see what happens.

For example, let's say that you're sitting comfortably across from me with your eyes closed and you're allowing your muscles to relax (***Let Go and Relax***) as you listen intently to my voice (***Focus on One Thing***). I'm repeating again and again the idea, "Your right arm is feeling warm, light, and comfortable." As you listen intently (***Take in Ideas***), you may eventually notice something interesting. Some people tell me that they feel a nice sensation in that arm while others describe seeing themselves lying on the beach and feeling the sun warming their arm. Still others just feel like they are calmly sitting in the chair. There are many ways that you can take in the ideas and enter a Trance.

"Can You Make Me Do Things Against My Will?"

This is a very anxiety-provoking question that a number of people have asked me. Another form of this question I've come across is: "Can the hypnotist put any idea into my mind and make me do things I don't want to do?" The answer is "No way, baby!" Since "All Hypnosis is Self-Hypnosis," you're in control of what goes into your mind. For example, let's say that you were sitting and relaxing in front of me with your eyes closed and you focused on my voice. Imagine that I said, "Your left arm is feeling comfortable." You'd probably take that idea in because most of us enjoy a good feeling in our body. But if I said, "You will get the urge to quack like a duck," I'll bet you'd open your eyes and tell me to "forget it, buddy," and stomp out of the room! Most people do not want to quack and would be insulted if you asked them. Again, you can't be forced to do anything just because I told you to.

It is possible for the hypnotist to offer you ideas that may shift some of your perception of a situation: For example, if she said, "You may feel a little warm," it's possible you may.

Stage Hypnosis and Clinical Hypnosis – The Differences

Usually, the above concerns come from people who know about or have seen Stage Hypnosis. The next few paragraphs will discuss the differences between Stage and Clinical (or Medical) Hypnosis.

- **Stage Hypnosis.** You might have seen a hypnotist at a fair, a bar, or a theater make people do all sorts of weird things in front of an audience. This is called "Stage Hypnosis" – or what I call "Hypno-tainment." It's the use of Hypnosis for entertainment purposes. These hypnotists are show-people who invite members of the audience up to their stage and eventually hypnotize them to do embarrassing and silly things (i.e., making animal sounds) – all to the delight and laughter of the crowd.

   How does the Stage Hypnotist get people to act that way? First, you have to observe what she does in the beginning of the show. They hypnotist will start by inviting to the stage "everyone who wants to get hypnotized." A rush of folks will make their way up there; each may have a different reason for coming up. Some of them want to prove that the hypnotist can't make them do anything; others are nervous and goaded by their friends to "try it," and still others just want to see what will happen. Next, the hypnotist will put them through a test. For example, she'll ask them to put their hands together in a prayer position with the fingers pointing to the ceiling. Then, she'll suggest to them that their hands are "stuck with glue and cannot be separated." When she invites them to try to separate their hands, some will not be able to do it. She'll then excuse the others and send them back to their seats. The remaining people are 1) willing to make fools out of themselves, and/or are 2) naturally very hypnotizable. They will do most anything the hypnotist will put them through for the sake of entertainment.

- **Clinical (Medical) Hypnosis.** The kind of Hypnosis I and my colleagues practice is not for entertainment purposes. It is called Clinical or Medical Hypnosis and its goal is to help you help yourself feel better and increase your mental and physical health. Unlike the people who want to act silly during Stage Hypnosis, you are interested in changing how your body feels and functions. The purpose of Clinical Hypnosis is to help you achieve your health goals by training you in techniques that will reduce the influence of chronic pain and Illness.

Hypnotic Choices – Online Digital Recording or Scripts

There are a number of options you can chose from to learn Self-Hypnosis. One very effective choice is to work with a qualified hypnotist and allow him or her to both guide you into trances and train you in how to do it yourself.[98] A second choice you can make is to allow me to train you…oh, but wait – you probably noticed that I am not physically sitting next to you right now. In that case, the next best thing I can do is provide you with a digital recording of my voice leading you through a hypnosis session. You can freely access one of these by going to my website (ComfortClinic.org).[99] You might also want to use any of the gazillion free recordings you'll find on sites like YouTube.

A third way to learn Hypnosis is to use one of the three Induction scripts provided in the Skill Box. This follows the next Story Box. Some of you may choose to use the Inductions yourself and spend time memorizing them, while others of you may prefer to ask a friend to guide you into a Hypnotic state by taking the role of "hypnotist" and reading the Induction to you. Both of these are fine.

Had a Trauma? – A Little WARNING!!

A number of you may have gone through a traumatic event or period of time in the past. Some who have this background may experience some anxiety when first practicing Hypnosis. If you have been traumatized by near-death experiences, war, child abuse, sexual assault, or other frightening occurrences, you should approach Hypnosis with a little caution. **If you have had serious trauma in your life, before you try using hypnosis on your own, please consult with a professional who is trained in Clinical Hypnosis (i.e., social worker, psychologist).** Your work with him or her can help you resolve some of the anxiety left over from previous traumatic experiences and enable you to eventually benefit from the use of hypnosis.

---

[98] Contact the "American Society of Clinical Hypnosis" or other Hypnosis organizations for referrals.
[99] Accessing Free Recording on ComfortClinic.org - on the Homepage click on the "More Information" link and then the "Resources" link. It's at the bottom of the page.

STORY BOX #34 - Gloria's Simple Hypnosis

Gloria suffered from inflamed ankles for many years. A mother of four she was determined to do something to reduce the fiery sensations she felt with each step. On the phone, she requested that I train her in Self-Hypnosis. I agreed and set an appointment for the next day. In thinking what I would do, I decided to guide her into a light Trance, then invite her to come out of it, and finally lead her into a second Trance during which I'd offer her "cooling" ideas that could ease the pain in her ankles. Sometimes, I'll direct people in and out of Trance because this will deepen their experience. Doing all of that was my plan.

The next day, I hypnotized Gloria into a relaxed state using a simple Count-Down Induction. I asked her to follow my count from "ten" down to "one" and, after I reached the last number, she could enjoy a pleasant experience. Ten minutes after she entered the Trance, I invited her back into the room with the intention of inviting her right back into Trance. However, I didn't need to do that because, to both our delights, she reported that her pain level had already reduced from an 8/10 to a 2/10! She was feeling much better despite the fact that I didn't suggest the cooling idea.

What Gloria did was allow this simple Trance state to raise her Comfort so high that she only felt 25% of the pain she had before practicing Hypnosis. What I learned was that when a person merely enters a hypnotic state this in itself can increase their comfort level by counting the numbers back from "one" up to "ten." I fully intended to hypnotize her again and use my "cooling" Trance technique but that was unnecessary now.

Skills of the Day (and Last Practice)

(A)
"Self-Hypnosis – Three Inductions"

Just as in Gloria's story, you may find that you'll feel relief simply by entering a Trance. What's surprising about this is the fact that you don't have to do anything fancy to directly elevate your Comfort level. If you are interested in learning three different Inductions that guide you into a Trance state, please use the next Skill Box.

RE-FOCUSING SKILL BOX #6 – "Self-Hypnosis – Three Inductions"

"Count Down Induction"

Step One - Quiet Place & Signal Timer. First, find a quiet place to sit. Choose a seat or recliner that will comfortably support your body. Recall that if you lie down, you might fall asleep. Use a timer that has a gentle alarm to signal you when you'd like to return.

Step Two - See, Hear or Feel the Numbers. Decide on which sense mode you'd like to use to follow your numbers down to a relaxed state. Some of you may want to hear the numbers quietly sounding in your mind; others will feel a sensation such as warm, heavy, or soft filling and surrounding your body as each number goes by. Still others of you may see things with your "mind's eye," such as seeing yourself drifting down a set of steps or imagine yourself floating down a gentle river while lying on a raft.

Step Three - Choose an Experience. Decide what you'd like to happen when you reach the number "one." Here is a short list of possibilities:
- **Repeat Count.** Continue the ten-to-one count again and again, moving deeper and deeper into relaxation with each repetition.
- **Happy Place.** Drift to a good place or an enjoyable experience you had in the past.
- **Floating.** Allow yourself to float in water or in the air, or settle into a quiet place of stillness like a pebble drifting down into a warm pond.

Step Four - Begin the Count-Down. Once you've decided on what you want to happen after the count, begin counting down from "ten" to "one" (quietly in your mind), and, once you reach "one," you can be there (i.e., the beach, or floating in the air). Remember, take your time; there's never a hurry.

Step Five - Returning. Finally, when you hear the alarm go off, follow your numbers back from "one" up to "ten." Or, you can return yourself to the room any way you'd like. Wait until you're fully awake before you take on any major tasks (i.e., like driving car).

"Deep Breathing Induction"

This induction is similar to Mantra Meditation in that you silently repeat a word each time your breath goes out. It differs because the word you use is actually a Hypnotic idea that brings you into a tranquil state (i.e., "Deeper").

Step One - Quiet Place & Signal Timer. First, find a quiet place to sit. Choose a seat or recliner that will comfortably support your body. Recall that if you lie down, you might fall asleep. Use a timer that has a gentle alarm to signal you to return to the room. Set it for the amount of time you want to be in Trance.

Step Two – "Deeply…"
- **Focus on Breath.** Begin to aim your attention at the feeling of the breath moving in and out of your belly (focus on chest if the belly hurts).
- **Repeating Words.**
  1) <u>On every inhale,</u> quietly in your mind, sound the word ***"Deeply"*** (you can also choose other neutral or positive words including *"Drifting," "Soothing," "Floating," or "Flowing"*).
  2) <u>On every exhale,</u> quietly in your mind, sound the word ***"Calm" or "Relaxed, or "Peaceful"*** (you can also choose other neutral or positive words such as *"Free," "Content," or "Open"*).
- **Continue to Float.** At some point, you'll enter a calm state and, if you'd like, you can either continue to focus on the breath and words, or you can switch your attention to focusing on the feeling of tranquility.

Step Three - Returning. Finally, when the alarm goes off, follow your numbers back by counting from "one" up to "ten." Or, you can return yourself to the room any way you'd like. Wait until you're fully awake and alert before you take on any major tasks (i.e., like driving car).

"Drifting"

This Re-Focusing Skill based on a relaxation technique first introduced by German psychiatrist Johannes Schulz in the 1930s. Very similar to Hypnosis, this Skill invites you to repeat one soothing idea over and over again in your mind. For example, as you relax and focus on your left arm, your inner voice might repeat the suggestion, "The left arm is feeling warm and comfortable." Those who use this technique have found that they drift into a very pleasant state of mind and body. Take twenty minutes now and follow the instructions in the steps below (or use the recording under "Resources" on my website ComfortClinic.org).

Step One - Quiet Place & Signal Timer. First, find a quiet place to sit. Choose a seat or recliner that will comfortably support your body. Use a timer that has a gentle alarm to signal you to return to the room.

Step Two – Choose a "Drifting" Phrase. The core of this technique involves your mentally repeating a soothing phrase over and over that relates to one of your limbs. Pick or create a phrase that sounds good to you. The following are some examples.
- "The right arm is warm, light, and comfortable"
- "The right arm is warm, heavy, and comfortable"
- "The right arm is cool, light, and soft"
- "The right arm is soft, warm, and easy"

Step Three – Brief Scan of the Body. As you sit or lie with your eyes closed, start at your feet and briefly notice each part of your body (skip those that are too uncomfortable to focus on).

Step Four – Practice Drifting. Once you finish Step Three, you can focus on your arms and legs by doing the following:
- **Repeat the Phrase.** Use the phrase you chose in Step Two and repeat it four or five times slowly in your mind as you concentrate on the part of the body it relates to. For example, if you repeat, "The right arm is warm, light and comfortable," focus your attention on the feeling in your right arm.
- **Pause and Drift.** After the repetitions of the phrase, pause for a quiet moment and notice what is going on in that limb. If you notice a pleasant feeling, drift with it for a while. Then, drift to the next arm or leg and repeat the phrase four or five times, slowly (i.e., "the left arm is warm, light, and comfortable"). Continue this process until you have completed all of your phrases.
- **Just Keep Drifting Until You Return.** Once you've finished your phrase sequence, allow yourself to drift with the relaxing calm until either your alarm goes off or you're ready to open your eyes and return to the room.

Example "Drifting" Script.

You might say in your mind the following words while "drifting" for about 30-to-60 seconds between each round of five repetitions:

- "The right arm is warm, light, and comfortable" (5x then Pause & Drift)
- "The left arm is warm, light, and comfortable" (5x then Pause & Drift)
- "The right leg is warm, light, and comfortable" (5x then Pause & Drift)
- "The left leg is warm, light, and comfortable" (5x then Pause & Drift)
- "The arms are warm, light, and comfortable" (5x then Pause & Drift)
- "The legs are warm, light, and comfortable" (5x then Pause & Drift)
- "The arm & legs are warm, light, & comfortable" (5x Pause & Drift)
- (Continue quietly, calmly drifting until you are ready to return)

Remember

➢ **Just Notice.** You don't have to force anything to happen; just follow the count, notice what happens and allow the Trance to unfold.

➢ **Re-Focusing.** If you get a visit from the thought "nothing is happening," let it go and continue to focus on what is happening.

➢ **Enjoy the Calm State.** At some point, you'll enter a calm state; feel free to stay there as long as you'd like, even after your alarm goes off.

HOMEWORK BOX
THIRD TRAINING DAY – WEEK 7

1. **One Hypnosis Skill.** Practice one of the Self-Hypnosis Inductions above.

2. **Rehearse Direct or Indirect Limit Setting in Your Imagination.** Review these Skills and imagine applying one to a difficult interaction you've had with an Annoying Person (see pages 298-301).

3. **Notice Positive Change.** In the days between now and the next Training Day, notice any large or small positive changes that enter your life and write them down. Ask yourself each day:

**"What happened today, large or small,
that I want to see more of in my life?"**

Week Eight – Comfort Skills Review & Seeing a New Future
Eight Week Basic Training

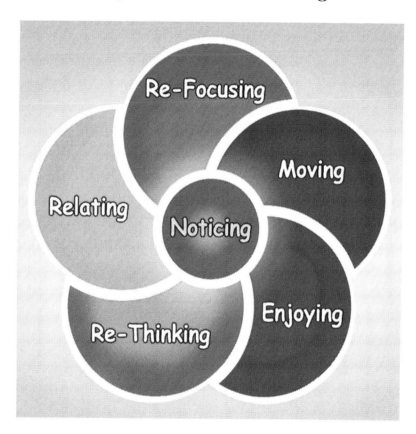

My Hope

I hope that the 8-Week Basic Training program has helped you to feel more comfortable despite the challenges that chronic pain has put you through. In this last weekly section, I'll review every Comfort Skill included in the eight weeks of training and introduce you to a couple more. Recall that the Skills are organized into six categories called Comfort Strategies. I represent these on the Comfort Wheel above. As this section unfolds, I'll present each Skill within its Comfort Strategy and also include the specific Pain Problems that they address.

WEEK EIGHT CONTENTS BOX
Noticing and Re-Focusing Strategies
First Training Day

1. The Skill Review
   A) Re-Focusing Skill
   B) *"I Want to See More of…"*
2. Solving Pain Problems with the Noticing Strategy
3. Solving Pain Problems with the Re-Focusing Strategy
4. Skill of the Day
   A) *"Comparison Questions"*
5. The Last Practice
   A) Re-Focusing Skill
6. Homework Box

Moving and Enjoying Strategies
Second Training Day

1. The Skill Review
   A) Re-Focusing Skill
   B) *"Comparison Question"*
2. Solving Pain Problems with the Moving Strategy
3. Solving Pain Problems with the Enjoying Strategy
4. The Last Practice
   A) Re-Focusing Skill
5. Homework Box

Re-Thinking and Relating Strategies
Third Training Day

1. The Skill Review
    A) Re-Focusing Skill
2. Solving Pain Problems with the Re-Thinking Strategy
3. Solving Pain Problems with the Relating Strategy
4. The Last Practice
    A) Re-Focusing Skill
5. Homework Box for the Rest of Your Life!

Noticing and Re-Focusing Skills
First Training Day – Week 8

(A)
Re-Focusing Skills

For at least 20 minutes, practice one Re-Focusing Skill (see list on page 338).

(B)
"I Want to See More of..."

Consult your Journal or digital disk, or review the last several days and answer the two questions below.

- **"What happened since the last Training Day, large or small, that I want to see more of in my life?"**
- **"What caused these things to happen?"**

Solving Pain Problems with the Noticing Strategy

The Noticing Strategy includes the four Skills described below. Two of them enable you to notice the "Negatives" that warn you about harmful events. These Skills help you avoid, reduce, or better tolerate pain flares and emotional upsets. The other two Noticing Skills open your eyes to some of the Positives in your life and help you notice desired improvements in your life.

Pain Problem #1 -
"Unpredictable Pain Flares and Emotional Distress"

Difficulties like pain flares and emotional upsets seem to come out of nowhere, leaving you feeling helpless and frustrated.

Noticing Skill Solutions – Negatives
Noticing Skill # 1 – "Revealing Triggers"

This Noticing Skill shows you how to reveal "**Triggers**," which are harmful occurrences that usually originate outside of you, in the physical or social world, or from an activity. A Trigger often sets off a bad mood or a pain flare (i.e., bright lights). (See page 148)

Noticing Skill # 2 – "Revealing First Signs"

This Skill trains you to notice **"First Signs,"** which take place inside your body and mind, such as muscle tension, negative thoughts and images, upset emotions, or a harmful habit like over-eating. These warn you that a pain flare or an upsetting event is coming. First Signs are often a response to a Trigger. Both Triggers and First Signs alert you to do something to prevent a painful episode (See page 149)

Pain Problem #8
"Missing the Good Things in Your Life"
Too often, pain and Misery dominate your attention so much that you may not notice pleasures, positive changes, and other good events that are already happening inside and around you.

Noticing Skill Solutions – Seeing Positives
Noticing Skill #3 – "I Want to See More of…"

"Positives" are satisfying changes that increase your comfort and well-being. This is the first of two Noticing Skills that shows you how to observe what's going well. It trains you to track the good things that arise in your life (even small ones). (See page 165)

Noticing Skill #4 – "Comparison Questions"

After completing part or all of the Trainings in this book, and practicing the Skills you've learned, many of you will notice some improvements happening in your daily life. The questions provided in this last Positive Noticing Skill help you see what is positively different now compared to where you were in the past. (See page 322)

Solving Pain Problems with the Re-Focusing Strategy

The Re-Focusing Strategy includes eight Skills that help you to develop your "concentration muscle" – to allow the pain to be there and redirect your attention towards neutral or pleasurable things. By doing this, you calm your nervous system and increase your feelings of Comfort and joy. This set of Skills empowers you to change three common Pain Problems.

Pain Problem #2
"Attention Hijacked by Pain and Stress"

Your attention becomes overly absorbed by pain as well as stress, anxiety, and/or other emotional upsets. This is because you have unknowingly allowed yourself to focus on these difficulties and your brain has grown used to directing its attention towards them.

Pain Problem #4 –
"Sadness, Worry, and Other Miserable Feelings"

You find little pleasure in life and often feel depressed, angry, worried, anxious, and/or bored. These feelings are often brought on by the uncomfortable sensations you feel in your body. These miseries make it difficult for you to feel pleasure or anything good.

Pain Problem #9 –
"Hypersensitive Nervous System"

Pain and stress have made your nervous system very sensitive to the pain signals traveling through it. In many cases, the brain has been altered by the ongoing pain and Misery experience, causing things that did not hurt in the past to hurt now. Also, what used to sting a little now stings a lot more.

Re-Focusing Skill Solutions
Re-Focusing Skill #1 – "Breath Count"

The title says it all – this Skill instructs you to count each exhale quietly in your mind. After you reach ten breaths, start over again with "one." Like the other Re-Focusing Skills, when you notice that you've gotten distracted by thoughts, sounds, or feelings, gently return your attention back to the breath and the count. (See page130.)

Re-Focusing Skill #2 – "Breath Massage"

This practice enables you to "massage" your body by imagining that your breath is flowing through each body part. As you focus intently on it, you may begin to feel like you're receiving a massage. (See page151.)

Re-Focusing Skill #3 – "Mantra/Breath Meditation"

The first of two Meditation techniques described in this book, "Mantra/Breath Meditation," involves your repeating a word (or Mantra) in your mind each time your breath moves (i.e., "calm," or "Relax"). This allows you to alter how your brain processes pain signals and it strengthens your ability to focus your attention. (See page 198.)

Re-Focusing Skill #4 – "Mindfulness Meditation/Thought Labeling"

This is one form of a powerful method to reduce suffering and raise your Comfort. It was introduced to the medical world by Dr. Jon Kabat-Zinn, a research scientist in the early 1980s. As you practice this style of Meditation, you allow distracting thoughts and feelings to "just be there" as you mentally label them and return to focus. Over time, distractions will bother you less, your mind and nervous system will become calmer, and your body will feel more at ease. (See page 226.)

Re-Focusing Skill #5 – "The Head Trip"

Daydreaming is a natural skill that we all use when we're bored or just want to fantasize about something. In a way, when you use your imagination to go on a "Head Trip," you can "leave your body" for a while and go on a little imaginary adventure. Once you return, your body may pleasantly surprise you. (See page 245.)

Re-Focusing Skill #6 – "Self-Hypnosis – Three Inductions"

Thre hypnotic techniques are offered as a way to invite you into a deep state of relaxation. (See page 311.)

Re-Focusing Skill #7 – "Positive Distraction –
The Fast and Slow Menus"

Research and common sense have shown that when you distract yourself you temporarily forget what you were experiencing in the moment. Positive Distractions may interrupt the pain, even for a little while. There are two forms of this Skill suggested on page 265.)

Re-Focusing Skill #8 – "Immerse in a Good Memory"

This Skill combines the internal concentration that characterizes Re-Focusing Skills with the pleasant feeling brought about by Enjoying Skills. It is the practice of replaying wonderful memories in your mind and fully re-experiencing and enjoying them. (See page 230.)

Skill of the Day

(A)
"Comparison Questions"

"Comparison Questions" *invite you to identify any positive changes that have occurred since you began practicing the Skills in this program (in either the Brief- or Eight-Week Training).* You might find it very interesting to discover what positive changes have developed over the time you have been practicing Comfort Skills. The questions in the Box below help you notice what your Comfort, mood, and activity levels are now compared to what they were before you started the Training. Because profound change often comes about gradually, you may more easily see it after a couple of months.

In the Noticing Skill Box #4, you will find a list of questions that can help you reveal what has changed since you began this program.

NOTICING SKILL BOX #4 –
"Comparison Questions"

Step One – Ask Yourself Comparison Questions. Each of the Comparison questions below define "the past" as any number of days, weeks, months, or years. Answer one or more of these questions. Perhaps you can create some of your own.

Step Two – Record Your Answers. Use your Journal or digital file to record your answers to the Comparison Questions you choose. You'll benefit by reviewing your answers regularly (i.e., 1x month).

The Questions

❖ Compared to the Past, What Positives Are Happening Now That Were Not Happening Back Then? (i.e., walk five minutes a day)

❖ What Negatives (i.e., flares, stress) Are Happening Less Now Compared to the Past?

❖ What Activities Are You Doing Now That You Were Not Able to Do in the Past?

❖ Are You Using Less Pain Medications Now Compared to the Past? If So, What Dose?

❖ What Daily Pain Level (where 10/10 is the worst), Are You Feeling Now Compared to the Past?

❖ Compared to the Past, How Much Better is Your Mood Today (where "0" is a very low mood and "10" is very high mood)?

❖ What Bad Habits Have Changed and How Much?

❖ How Much Time Do You Presently Spend on Negative Thinking Compared to the Past?

❖ Compared to the Past, What Comfort Skills Are You Practicing Regularly Now That You Were Not Doing in the Past? How Much More Effective Are They Now than in the Past?

The Last Practice
Re-Focusing Skills

For 20 minutes practice one Re-Focusing Skill on page 338.

HOMEWORK BOX
FIRST TRAINING DAY – WEEK 8

1. **Daily Re-Focusing Skill.** Practice one or more of these Skills listed above for at least 20 minutes a day (see page 338).

2. **Comparison Questions.** Use the Skills Box above to ask yourself a Comparison question or two and record your answers.

Moving and Enjoying Skills
Second Training Day – Week 8

The Skill Review

(A)
Re-Focusing Skills

For 20 minutes, practice one Re-Focusing Skill (see page 338).

(B)
"Comparison Questions"

Ask yourself a Comparison Question you have not used yet and record your answer in your Journal or digital file (see page 323).

Solving Pain Problems with the Moving Strategy

The Moving Strategy includes eight Skills that empower you to move through four activities: 1) Goal Setting, 2) Moving the Body, 2) Sleep and Rest, and 4) Pain Flare Planning. These Skills help you to avoid four Pain Problems associated with these activities.

Pain Problem #10
"No Positive Future in Sight"

Too often, when chronic pain comes, he and Depression like to convince you that you no longer have a happy future. It's easy to believe this if you can no longer do your job or carry out daily activities. You might feel like there is nothing good to look forward to.

Moving Yours Goals
Moving Skill #1 – "Set a Goal, Create a Future"

Often, when chronic pain or Depression comes along, you might Under-Do your activity by lying around too much and unintentionally making your body worse over time. When you set a goal, (i.e., social, exercise, work), you're telling Depression and Pain that you <u>do</u> have a future. You'll also return to a balanced level of activity and build a new life, goal by goal. There is no rush – the practice works best when you go at a slow, steady pace by taking "Baby Steps" – that is, move one small step at a time. (See pages 133 & 138.)

Pain Problem #11
"Over-Doing"

You find yourself drawn into activities that lead to pain flares, misery, and/or exhaustion. This often occurs when you Over-Do ("OD") your activity or engage in something that automatically flares the pain (i.e., lifting heavy objects)

Moving the Body
Moving Skill #2 – "Pay as You Go"

Many people in pain tend to Over-Do their activities beyond what their body can comfortably handle. If you want to avoid pain flares brought on by over-exertion and high stress, use this Skill to adjust a task so that it fits your body and increases Comfort. (See page 169.)

Moving Skill #3 – "The Payment Plan."

For those of you who believe that Over-Doing a certain activity is worth the pain flare you'll get, there is still an option you can use to effectively ride out the increased discomfort. The three components of this Skill will enable you to more easily handle a pain flare and, in the end, you may ride it out more comfortably than in the past. (See page 176.)

Pain Problem #3
"Poor Sleep and Rest at Night"

You feel exhausted and achy in the morning because you had a difficult time falling and/or staying asleep. In part, this is because you're dealing with many distractions, physical and psychological, that keep you awake.

Sleep and Rest
Moving Skill #4 – "Day Skills for Night Sleep"

When you use some or all of this collection of techniques during the day, you can improve your ability to sleep at night. (See page 184.)

Moving Skill #5 – "Rest in the Bed"

This is one of two powerful Skills you can use if you have a difficult time falling and/or staying asleep. When you follow its three steps, you can feel more rested in the morning, even if you did not sleep that night. (See page 189.)

Moving Skill #6 – "Working Back to Bed"

If you find it difficult to stay in bed at night when you can't sleep, this second night-time Skill gives you a work assignment that can lead you back to a bed of sleep or rest. (See page 188.)

Pain Problem #7
"Underprepared for Pain Flares"

When pain flares come, you may feel unprepared to handle them and that adds to the hurt and upset. When you're caught off guard, you're likely to feel helplessness and panic.

Moving Through a Pain Flare
Moving Skill #7 – "Flare Planning in Sets of Three"

When pain flares come along, this Moving Skill helps you to more effectively ride them out. It will instruct you on how to set up a plan to deal with future increases in pain. (See page 270.)

Moving Skill #8 – "Two Bottles of Comfort"

There are two bottles you can use to help you handle a pain flare. The first, "The Skill Bottle," is a device that helps you to recall those Skills that help you deal with chronic pain. The second, "The Flare Bottle," offers you a safe way to use short-acting opiate and other pain medications to help you increase your Comfort during a pain flare. Most people in pain who use pain medications are very responsible in the way they use these drugs. However, there are times when the medicine does not touch the sharpness of the pain. It's during those moments that many folks feel the need to take more than prescribed on the bottle. In consultation with your doctor, you may find that using this Skill will enable you to use your medication more effectively (See page 273.)

Solving Pain Problems with the Enjoying Strategy

The Enjoying Strategy includes five Skills, all designed to help you raise your mood in order to increase your Comfort level. There are three kinds of Enjoying Skills – 1) "Enjoying Right Now," which raises your mood in the moment, 2) "Positive U-Turn," which helps you to turn away from something Negative and turn toward something positive, and 3) "Cultivating Positive Qualities," which directs you to identify and strengthen your Positive Qualities (i.e., gratitude).

Pain Problem #2
"Attention Hijacked by Pain and Stress"

Your attention becomes overly absorbed by pain as well as stress, anxiety, and/or other emotional upsets. This is because you have unknowingly allowed yourself to focus on these difficulties and the brain has grown used to directing its attention towards them.

Pain Problem #4 –
"Sadness, Worry, and Other Miserable Feelings"

You find little pleasure in life and often feel depressed, angry, worried, anxious, and/or bored. These feelings are often brought on by the uncomfortable sensations you feel in your body. These miseries make it difficult for you to feel anything good.

Pain Problem #9 –
"Hypersensitive Nervous System"

Pain and stress have made your nervous system very sensitive to the pain signals traveling through it. In many cases, the brain has been altered by the ongoing pain and Misery experience, causing things that did not hurt in the past to hurt now. Also, what used to sting a little now hurts a lot more.

Enjoying Right Now
Enjoying Skill # 1 – "Laughing"

This Skill invites you to bring more Laughter into your daily life. There is ample medical and psychological evidence that laughter raises your Comfort level and contributes to your general health (laugh right now and see what happens). As long as laughter does not irritate the part of your body that hurts, you'll notice that when you use this Skill you'll feel lighter, happier and more at ease. (See page 158.)

Enjoying Skill # 2 – "Doing Fun"

Similar to Laughing, this lifestyle practice raises your mood and makes it easier to tolerate physical pain. Pleasurable activity does not have to be expensive or even strenuous. The important point of this Skill is to increase the times in your life when you are enjoying yourself, even a little. (See Chapter Eight, Week Two, Second Training Day.)

Positive U-Turn
Enjoying Skill #3 – "Counter a Negative with a Positive"

This Enjoying Skill helps you to "snatch joy from the mouth of Misery." When you're in a painful situation, you may often feel like you are trapped and that there's no escape. Use this Skill to counter a Negative that's in your face and you'll be happy you did!. (See page 168.)

Cultivating Positive Qualities
Enjoying Skill #4 – "Write a Gratitude Letter"

A "Positive Quality" is a strongly held, life affirming purpose, value, and ability that defines your character. Scientists have identified twenty-four of these.[100] One of the most powerful Positive Qualities is "Gratitude." When you engage in it, you have the potential to develop a sense of appreciation for life (something very difficult to do when chronic pain shows up).[101] (See page 253.)

Enjoying Skill #5 – "Filling a 'Good Stuff' Journal"

Another way to cultivate your Quality of Gratitude is to keep a Journal dedicated to the "Good Stuff" in your life. (See page 254.)

The Last Practice
Re-Focusing Skills

For 20 minutes, practice one Re-Focusing Skill from the list on page 388.

---

[100] See Christopher Peterson and Martin Seligman's book, "Character Strengths and Virtues: A Handbook and Classification" 2004.
[101] See Robert Emmons' book, "Thanks."

HOMEWORK BOX
SECOND TRAINING DAY – WEEK 8

1. **Remember Your Basic Training Goal? – "How Close Did You Get?"** Ask yourself how close you got to the goal you set in the first Training Week. Did you reach it or did you have to adjust it some? What were the obstacles and how did you get past them? If there were obstacles that slowed you down, how would you get past them today? What new goals would you like to pursue now? (Even if you didn't set a goal → ask yourself, "What is positively different in my life today?") See the Goal-Setting Skill on pages 133 &138 to develop new goals.

2. **Moving Skills for Sleep**. If sleep is still difficult, review and practice the sleep skills (see pages 184-188).

3. **Spending Your Comfort Time.** Review how you're protecting yourself from Over-Doing and Under-Doing and the pain flares they cause. Review these powerful Skills:
   - **"Pay As You Go,"** or **"The Payment Plan"** can protect your body from flares set off by Over-Doing (see pages 169 & 176).

4. **"Fun and Laughter."** Do something you enjoy at least once a day. If you don't know what to do for fun, watch something that makes you laugh! (See pages 158 & 162.)

5. **Make a Positive U-Turn**. Choose a difficult situation you've encountered in the past and consider how you'd better cope with it using the "Counter a Negative with a Positive" Skill (see page 239).

6. **Cultivate Your Positive Qualities.** Choose and cultivate at least one or more of your Positive Qualities (see pages 253 & 254).

Re-Thinking and Relating Skills
Third Training Day – Week Eight

The Skill Review

(A)
Re-Focusing Skills

For 20 minutes, practice one Re-Focusing Skill from the list on page 338.

Solving Pain Problems with the Re-Thinking Strategy

The Re-Thinking Strategy includes four Skills that fall into two categories. The first Skill enhances your ability to remember. The remaining three Skills help you reduce the Negative Thoughts that often accompany chronic pain. They show you how to change low moods, anxiety, and worry by catching and neutralizing these Negative Thoughts.

Pain Problem #12
"Poor Memory"

Your memory and concentration are compromised by many factors – pain, medication, low moods, anxiety, stress, and poor sleep.

Re-Thinking Memory
Re-Thinking Skill #1 – "Look in the Book."

Since memory loss and poor concentration are common in people who are in chronic pain, you will find it most useful to take on this Re-Thinking Skill. (See page 205.)

Pain Problem #5
"Negative Thoughts"

You're plagued by negative thoughts that relentlessly drive you into emotional distress and harmful habits. This is because your situation often brings on these thoughts and you unknowingly follow them down the road to miserable places. Both of these tent to increase pain

---

Re-Thinking Negative Thoughts
Re-Thinking Skill #2 – "See it Coming"

Pain, Depression, and other "Bad Characters" often send Negative Thoughts into your mind when you feel emotionally vulnerable and physically uncomfortable. Thoughts like "My life is over" or "I'm just a cripple" will usually bring your mood down or worry you and this causes the Pain and Misery to raise. This Re-Thinking Skill shows you how to catch these thoughts before they catch you, enabling you to stand up to them, build your self-control, and raise up your mood. (See page 215.)

Re-Thinking Skill #3 – "Re-Mind Yourself About the Truth"

Just like a number of lawyers and politicians, Negative Thoughts lie to you. Untruths such as "you're a loser" or "you are a lazy burden on everyone" can really hurt you if you believe them. This Skill reminds you to consider what is true in the face of such harmful thoughts. (See page 218.)

Re-Thinking Skill #4 – "Talk Back and Step Aside"

When Negative Thoughts bug you, you'll find it very helpful to "talk back" to them in your mind. When you do this and combine it with "stepping aside" (distracting yourself), you'll weaken that thought and improve your mood. This prevents additional pain and suffering that often accompanies people in pain who fall into depression or anxiety. (See page 220.)

Solving Pain Problems with the Relating Strategy

The Relating Strategy includes seven Skills described below. Two of them advise you on how to connect and re-connect to good people, and five of them help you to calmly and firmly set limits on "Annoying People," those who criticize, manipulate, and irritate you.

Pain Problem #13
"Isolation and Loneliness"

You feel isolated and miserably alone, and/or you're terribly bored and this adds to your suffering and discomfort. This often occurs when you avoid good people or when the friends you thought you had abandon you.

Relating with Good People
Relating Skill #1 –
Build New Relationships with Old Friends and Family

Many people in pain are socially isolated and feel very, very lonely. This Relating Skill shows you how to renew old relationships with the good people in your life. Most social and health scientists agree that positive relationships lead to positive feelings and physical health. (See page 260.)

Relating Skill #2 – How to Meet New Friends

New relationships also increase your joy. Some of you may have been abandoned by some of your old "friends." When this happens, you discover who your real friends are. The goal of this second Relating Skill is to help you explore new people who might turn into true friends. (See page 262.)

Pain Problem #6
"Distressed by Annoying People"

There are people in your life that you relate with regularly. Some of them you may deeply know and love. Unfortunately, at times, they hurt you with their criticizing, manipulating, or intimidating words and actions. Sometimes, you may believe their hurtful words and give in to their unreasonable demands.

Dealing with Annoying People Directly
Relating Skill #3 – "The C.A.L.M. Nice Guy Approach"

We all have "Annoying People" in our lives. These are usually loved ones or co-workers who annoy you from time to time or bother you about a particular issue (i.e., spending money, use of pain medication). There are also "Seriously Annoying People" – those who irritate you most every day (i.e., a sarcastic, controlling spouse). Whether they bother you a little or a lot, the result is the same – you feel stressed out, miserable, and pained. When you set an effective limit on their behavior, especially on their hurtful words, your life can feel much better. The "C.A.L.M. Nice Guy Approach is one direct method to say "No!" to an Annoying Person. (See page 290.)

Relating Skill #4 – "The C.U.T. Tough Guy Approach"

This is another direct way to say "No!" to an Annoying Person. The "C.U.T. Tough Guy Approach" shows you how to immediately get firm with those who don't respect your reasonable requests. (See Chapter Eight, Week Seven, First Training Day.)

Dealing with Annoying People Indirectly
Relating Skill #5 – "One Down Duck Down"

Some situations call for a more indirect approach to say "No!" to the abuses of Annoying People. The "One Down Duck Down" is quite effective in stopping the verbal abuse and preventing yourself from getting defensive. (See page 297.)

Relating Skills #6 – "Disarm Them in the F.O.G."

This technique gives your tormentors an indirect consequence for the irritation they cause you. Often, that will dissuade them from bothering you. (See page 298.)

Relating Skills #7 – "Distracted Listening"

Don't you wish you could find a way to avoid listening to an Annoying Person spouting his or her hurtful, irritating words? This Skill shows you how to indirectly set a limit on their Toxic Talk by getting distracted on purpose (See page 301.)

The Last "Last Practice"

Re-Focusing Skills

For 20 minutes, practice one Re-Focusing Skill listed on page 338.

THE LAST HOMEWORK BOX
For the Rest of Your Life!

See "Appendix A" (on page 388) to locate the following Skills:

1. **Re-Focusing Skill Practice.** Every day for at least 20 minutes, use any of the Re-Focusing Skills you learned in the Training.

2. **Create Social Connections.** Take a few more steps towards spending time with good people. If you already do this, do a little more. Use some of the Relating Skill Boxes to help you do this.

3. **Imagine Setting a Direct Limit.** Review the two Skills that help you deal with Annoying People directly, then, imagine applying one to a person who irritates you. Later, apply it to real situation.

4. **Imagine Setting an Indirect Limit.** Review the two Skills that help you to indirectly say "No!" to an Annoying Person then imagine applying one to a difficult interaction you've had with him or her. Later, apply it to real situation.

5. **"One Fun a Day."** Do something you enjoy at least once a day.

6. **Laugh Your Head Off.** Watch funny movies, little kids, TV sit-coms, dogs, online shows, or other sources to laugh every day for at least 30 minutes (See the "Funny Box" for Youtube selections on page 161).

7. **Make a Positive U-Turn.** Either imagine or choose a difficult situation and consider how you can turn it around by using the "Counter a Negative with a Positive" Skill.

8. **Remember to Remember.** Create or add to a Memory Book and review your daily schedule by looking in the book every morning to improve your memory.

9. **Re-Think Negative Thoughts.** Use Re-Thinking Skills #'s 2, 3, and 4 to change the Negative Thoughts that bother you.

10. **"Set a Goal, Create a Future**." Notice how close you got to the goal you set at the beginning of this Training Course Did you reach it? Did you have to adjust it some? What were the obstacles and how did you get past them? What new goals do you want to pursue next? (See pages 133 & 138.)

11. **Looking for Positives.** At the end of each day or week, ask yourself these two questions:
    ▪ *"What's been happening, large or small, that I want to see more of in my life?"*
    ▪ *"What caused these things to happen?"*

12. **Moving Skills for Sleep**. Review and practice the sleep and rest Skills.

13. **Spending Your Comfort Time.** Review how you're protecting yourself from Over-Doing and Under-Doing and the pain flares they cause by practicing: **"Pay As You Go,"** or **"The Payment Plan"** to protect your body and better ride out pain flares set off by Over-Doing.

14. **Noticing Triggers & First Signs of Trouble.** Continue catching the Triggers and the First Signs that warn you about approaching pain flares or emotional upsets. Once you identify them, use some of the other Skills to increase your Comfort and reduce Misery and flares.

15. **Comparison Questions.** Every month or so, ask yourself one or more of the Comparison Questions to help you notice positive changes

Appendices

Appendix A ~ Comfort Menu – Finding the Strategies and Skills

As you'll soon learn in more detail, you can use "Comfort Skills" to increase the Comfort in of your body and mind. Each of the thirty-six Comfort Skills included in this book are listed here under its corresponding Comfort Strategy category. Each also includes the page number where you can find it.

First Comfort Strategy – Noticing

The first of two Skills shows you how to identify "Negatives" that either set off or warn you about a coming pain flare or emotional upset. Two other Noticing Skills shine your awareness on "Positives."

Noticing Skills – Negatives

Noticing Skills – Positives

Second Comfort Strategy – Re-Focusing Skills

This set of Skills helps you redirect your attention away from pain and towards something neutral or pleasant. Each Re-Focusing practice potentially relaxes your mind and body and reduces stress and pain sensitivity in your nervous system.

Third Comfort Strategy – Moving Skills

This strategy shows you how to comfortably and effectively move through four important events in your life: Goal Setting, Moving the Body, Sleep and Rest, and Pain Flares.

Goal Setting

Moving the Body

Sleep and Rest

Moving Through a Pain Flare

Fourth Comfort Strategy – Enjoying Skills

Enjoying Skills generate pleasure, raise your mood, and increase your calm, all causing pain to take a back seat in your life.

Enjoying Right Now

Positive U-Turn

Cultivating Positive Qualities

Fifth Comfort Strategy – Re-Thinking Skills

It's clear that low moods, anxiety, stress, and pain-focusing are often brought on by Negative Thoughts. This Strategy includes three Skills that enable you to prevent bad thoughts from taking you to places you don't want to go. It also includes a Skill to improve your memory.

Re-Thinking Memory

Re-Thinking Negative Thoughts

Sixth Comfort Strategy -Relating Skills

Your physical and emotional comfort is profoundly impacted by your interactions with people. Pain and Misery levels rise when you isolate yourself from good people, argue a lot, or give in to the criticisms or manipulations of annoying people. These Skills show you how to connect with good people and set firm limits on annoying people.

Relating with Good People

Dealing with Annoying People Directly

Dealing with Annoying People Indirectly

Appendix B ~ "Learn/Abouts" – A List of Twenty-Three

In this appendix, you can locate each Learning About by turning to its corresponding page number.

Appendix C ~ Story Box List

Locate each Story Box by turning to its corresponding page number.

Appendix D ~ Info Box List

Appendix E ~ Comfort Killers – Twelve Harmful Habits to Avoid

A **"Harmful Habit"** *is an action you regularly engage in that hurts your health and well-being.* Although you will often perform these Habits on purpose, at times it may seem like they happen on their own. Sadly, when you engage in them, they increase Misery and Pain. This is why I also call them "Comfort Killers" (a quick list is on the next page).

In this Appendix, I'll describe each Harmful Habit and how it kills Comfort. The twelve Habits are divided into two categories defined by where they occur:

1. *External Habits take place between you and the people and situations around you.* For example, if you engaged in the Habit of "Doing for Everyone but Yourself," you'd over-focus on the needs of the people around you to the exclusion of your own.

2. *Internal Habits are those that take place inside of you.* For example, "Pain Focusing" directs your attention towards the parts of the body that hurt. It also causes you to ruminate on negative expectations and worry.

Eight External Harmful Habits
Harmful Habit #1 - "Over-Doing and Under-Doing"

People who engage in this Habit either Over-Do or Under-Do their activity level. Some people-in-pain take on too much activity and others do very little. On the one hand, if you engage in Over-Doing, you might clean the house for several hours at a time or lift too much weight. This can stress your mind and body and set off a pain flare. On the other hand, if you Under-Do by lying down or sitting around a lot, your body will feel the stiffness and misery of searing pain. In addition, when you fail to move your body enough (i.e., by watching hours and hours of bad TV), you can become vulnerable to emotional difficulties like Depression and Anxiety. As you apply Moving Skills to your life, you'll learn how to develop a balanced, comfortable level of activity that will help you avoid this Harmful Habit.

Harmful Habit #2 - "Doing for Everyone but Yourself"

When I describe this Habit in my Workshop, I usually project a photo of a mother dog lying on her side and nursing about a dozen puppies. When you are willing to give and give and give to other people, but not to yourself, everyone is very willing to suck the life out of you. This causes exhaustion, tension, and eventual pain flares. When you use Relating and Moving Skills to say "No" to some of this over-giving, and reduce your Over-Doing, you take the first step towards self-care and increased Comfort.

INFO BOX #24 -
"The Comfort Killers" - Twelve Harmful Habits

External Habits

1. Over-Doing and Under-Doing

2. Doing for Everyone but Yourself

3. Taking in Toxic-Talk (from Annoying Others)

4. Raging, Arguing, and Fighting

5. Ineffective Complaining

6. Self-Isolating from Good People

7. Fruitlessly Seeking the Cure

8. Avoiding Comfort Skills

Internal Habits

9. Pain Focusing

10. Following Negative Thoughts and Moods

11. Yearning for the Old Body

12. Stressing and Panicking

Harmful Habit #3 - "Taking in Toxic-Talk" (from Annoying Others)

"Taking in Toxic Talk from (Annoying Others")?....I know – it's a bit of a tongue twister. However, it's an accurate title for this Harmful Habit. To say it bluntly, some of you are willing to take in a lot of "crap" from people in your life who often criticize, manipulate, and intimidate you. When you allow this to happen, it brings on guilt, depression, rage, and worry. These destructive feelings raise up Misery and Pain levels. When you use Relating Skills, you will learn how to stop listening to the harsh words of Annoying People, spend more time with Good People, and feel a whole lot better.

Harmful Habit #4 - "Raging, Arguing, and Fighting"

This one is obvious – when you immerse yourself in anger, or verbally or physically fight with someone, you'll end up feeling lousy. Rage comes in many forms: You might pace back and forth and yell at the wall about how pissed off you are; you might sit and stew quietly in muscle tension or you replay the same angry thoughts over and over in your mind; or you might even turn your frustration into a fist fight. Sometimes, this leads you into trouble with spouses (who may kick you out of the relationship), or with the police (who will imprison you). Whether it's feuding with the family, growling at your doctor, or shouting at another driver on the road – arguing and fighting will jack up the pain. Using some of the Re-Focusing and Relating Skills will help bring calm back into your life and show you how to resolve conflict more peacefully. In other words, "Don't get mad, get even" (balanced and calm).

Harmful Habit #5 - "Ineffective Complaining"

Sometimes called "whining or kvetching," this Habit gets you nowhere and only brings you Misery. For example, you may find yourself in the middle of a "Pity Party" where you focus on all the losses you've had since the disease or injury brought pain and limitation into your life. If you choose to wallow in it you might feel a whole lot more pain, sadness, and stress. Also, people around you may want to avoid you if they hear too much of this kind of complaining.

All complaining is not bad – only Ineffective Complaining. You can engage in "Effective Complaining" and gain a lot of benefit from it. What is this? It is complaining that is short-lived and leads you to problem-solve your difficulties. Re-Thinking and Re-Focusing Skills can help you let go of Ineffective Complaining.

Harmful Habit #6 - "Self-Isolating from Good People"

It is very understandable that many of you may not feel like spending much time with people. Maybe you've been hurt by some of them or you tire of their constant questions (i.e., "How do you feel?) Perhaps you just don't have the energy or desire to talk these folks. It is a good thing to avoid people who are annoying you – IE, when they criticize, guilt-trip, argue with, and take advantage of you. Similarly, it's probably also healthier to stay away from people who are very negative or even dangerous. However, when you hang out with **Good People,** you get the opposite experience. Time spent with them on the phone or face-to-face can increase your Comfort level through a combination of positive distraction, social support, and a happier mood.

Actually, you are not really isolated when you practice the Habit of Self Isolation. No. You'll be hanging out with unsavory characters who are no fun to be with – Chronic Pain, Rage, Depression, and Anxiety. Relating Strategies can help you to move away from them and to draw closer to a positive social life with Good People.

STORY BOX #35 - Howard's 50th

Howard's life had not been the same since his neck surgery failed to significantly reduce the pain. Nearing his 50th birthday, Howard felt so depressed and hopeless that he avoided even phone contact with his close friends. He'd stay at home watching TV and feeling worse. Sadly, he was engaging in the Harmful Habit of "Self-Isolating from Good People." Eventually, he was willing to talk with me on the phone and, in time, he decided to stop this Habit by using the Re-Thinking and Relating Strategies. These helped him to move away from helpless and guilty thoughts and to return to some of the social times he used to have with his supportive friends. This, in turn, raised his mood and he felt a whole lot better. Later, to his joyful amazement, his friends threw him a surprise 50th birthday party!

Harmful Habit #7 - "Fruitlessly Seeking the Cure"

Here is the sad truth: Aside from a few exceptions, there is no cure for the conditions that cause chronic pain. There is no surgery, no Epidural, no Chiropractic adjustment, no Morphine Pump or other medical procedure, and no pill that will make it all go away. Even the "spinal stimulator" has been found to cause a number of medical complications for people. I'm sorry, I wish this were not true. I only tell you this in the hope that you'll stop "Fruitlessly Seeking the Cure." It does not exist. If you practice this Habit, it will empty your savings, put you through useless or minimally effective medical procedures, and cause you a lot of frustration and disappointment. Instead, you can use a number of Comfort Strategies , and your own resources, to move on with your life.

Harmful Habit #8 - "Avoiding Comfort Skills"

When you learn Skills, or use your own ways to increase your Comfort level, and you decide not to practice them, you'd be following the Harmful Habit of "Avoiding Comfort Skills." Helpless thoughts may stop some of you from using the Skills (i.e., "Nothing will help me feel better"). Some of you may not believe that anything short of a pill, injection or surgery will make a real difference in your body. As this book advocates, when you take certain actions in your life, you will begin to make the changes that modern medicine (or even alternative medicine) cannot. Others of you may acknowledge that the Skills would be helpful but you have a hard time "getting into the habit of practicing." All this is avoidance and will kill any potential Comfort you can get from practicing the Skills. When you approach the use of Comfort Skills with the intention to just "Do it to Do it" you will begin to slowly (and sometimes quickly) gain some well-deserved Comfort.

Four Internal Harmful Habits
Harmful Habit #9 - "Pain Focusing"

When you give more of your conscious awareness to pain than is necessary to take care of yourself, you may fall into the Harmful Habit of "Pain Focusing." If you direct most of your attention, along with negative expectations, towards the parts of the body that hurt, you may unintentionally kill your Comfort. You might even find yourself obsessing on uncomfortable feelings in the present, replaying memories of painful moments in the past, and anxiously ruminating on more hurt in the future.

Pain is a pretty persuasive attention-getter. To counter it, and the temptation to over-focus on it, you can use Re-Focusing and Enjoying Skills that show you how to direct your attention towards neutral and pleasurable sensations.

Harmful Habit #10 - "Following Negative Thoughts and Moods"

For most of you, before the pain came along, negative thoughts like "My life is over" or "I'm such a cripple" were not bouncing around in your mind very much, if at all. You also didn't focus a great deal on negative moods such as depression, anxiety, anger, or guilt. Now, many of you are seriously pestered by low thoughts and moods. What's really bad about this is that when you habitually follow negative thoughts and moods they lead you to more negative thoughts and moods! This also raises your physical discomfort. Re-Focusing, Re-Thinking, and Enjoying Skills can help you to change this.

Harmful Habit #11 - "Yearning for the Old Body"

By "Old Body," I'm referring to how your body felt before the pain came along. In that body, you could do many things with little discomfort or concern that you were going to hurt yourself or get a pain flare. Today, you have a "New Body," one that experiences chronic pain. When you get into the habit of "Yearning for the Old Body" you end up spending a lot of time either wishing you had your Old Body or feeling sad that you don't. This brings on a lot of disappointment and upset.

People who engage in this Harmful Habit are like poor drivers who constantly look in the rear-view mirror. Sure, they can see what's behind them, but they won't be able to move forward very well. In addition, people who put a lot of effort into Yearning for the Old Body never look forward to the possible things they can do with their New Body. This yearning for the Old Body knocks out any potential Comfort you could feel <u>now</u> or in the future because you're too busy pining over the way you lived in the past. As with Harmful Habit Number Ten, you can benefit by using Re-Focusing, Re-Thinking, and Enjoying Strategies to help free you from obsessing on the past and empower you to move towards a better future.

Harmful Habit #12 - "Stressing and Panicking"

You probably know that when you get into the Habit of Stressing and Panicking, the resulting surge of nervous energy will over stimulate your brain and nervous system and the pain will intensify. You also become increasingly hypersensitive to pain and that adds to the stress and panic. It's a vicious cycle. Comfort cannot last long in the face of this Habit. When you use Re-Focusing, Enjoying, and Re-Thinking Skills, this Habit begins to fade away.

Final Note – Changing Harmful Habits

Some of you already know what your Harmful Habits are. Others of you may have discovered them after reading this Appendix. If you're still unclear as to what Harmful Habits you may have, you can ask some of your close loved ones to help you. Sometimes an outside opinion from a caring friend or family member can reveal a lot. They might also provide you important information and insights that you can't see by yourself. Once you know what your Harmful Habits are, use the Skills in this book to change them.

Appendix F ~ Glossary of Definitions

Action Idea: A concept that you can act on.

Acute Pain: The physical discomfort produced by an injury or disease that eventually fades away once the underlying medical condition heals.

Allodynia: This occurs when physical sensations that didn't hurt in the past now become irritating (i.e., a light touch on the hand).

Ally: A person (or even a skill or action) that helps you stand up to an opponent or problem.

Annoying People: Individuals you know (and may love) whose behavior and words make you feel uncomfortable and upset.

Catastrophizing: A style of thinking which convinces you that events and situations are much worse than they really are.

Chronic Pain: A long-term, and often constant, level of pain regularly punctuated by sharp increases in discomfort ("pain flares").

Comfort: Combines a positive emotional state and optimistic mind-set that can include joy, peace, calm satisfaction, and pleasure – it's the opposite of Misery.

Comfort Skills: A collection of activities, exercises and techniques that empower you to reduce Misery and increase your Comfort level.

Comfort Strategies: Six categories of Comfort Skills that help you to increase Comfort and solve a set of problems brought on by pain-related problems.

Comfort Time: The amount of time and energy that you can spend doing activities comfortably.

Comparison Questions: These questions invite you to identify any positive changes that have occurred since you began practicing the Skills from the program (in either the Brief or Eight-Week training).

Daydreaming on Purpose: The intentional use of your imagination to have a desired experience.

Doctor Care Only: This common approach to chronic pain directs you to spend lots of your time passively receiving treatment from medical or other healthcare experts in a desperate effort to avoid pain.

Enjoying Strategy: The practice of raising your mood, positively coping with upsetting situations, and strengthening your positive qualities and sense of personal meaning.

First Signs: Your initial responses to a Trigger, these take place inside your body and mind and warn you that a pain flare or emotional upset is coming. For example, a small tension in your shoulder or worry thoughts.

Goal: An activity or experience that moves you towards a new, desirable future.

Gratitude: Is a positive Quality that fills your heart with feelings of appreciation and thankfulness towards a person or situation.

Harmful Habit: An action you regularly engage in that hurts your health and well-being.

Hyperalgesia: Occurs when small pains feel like big ones (i.e., a small finger prick that feels like a stabbing knife).

Meditation: This includes "…a family of techniques which have in common a conscious attempt to focus attention in a non-analytical way and an attempt not to dwell on discursive, ruminating thought."[102] Simply, Meditation is the practice of directing your attention and letting go of distractions such as thoughts, feelings, and sounds.

Mindfulness Meditation: The practice of noticing and accepting, in each moment, your thoughts, feelings, and bodily sensations and the surrounding environment while you let go of your tendency to judge or think about them. The primary focus is on what is going on in your mind.

Misery: Combines a distressed emotional state with a negative mind-set that can include stress, depression, guilt, rage, and anxiety – it's the opposite of Comfort.

---

[102] See "Meditation: Classic and Contemporary Perspectives," edited by Deane Shapiro, Jr & Roger Walsh.

Moving Strategy: The practice of moving comfortably and confidently through four tasks which are common to people-in-pain: Goal Setting, Moving the Body, Sleep and Rest, and Pain Flare Planning.

Negatives: Events that either set off or warn you that a pain flare or emotional upset is on the way.

Negative Thought: Any idea, belief, point of view, judgment, or mental image that increases your misery when you make it your focus of attention.

New Body: The state your body is in after chronic pain came along.

Noticing Strategy: The practice of making yourself aware of the positive and negative events that occur in your daily life with the intention of increasing the first and decreasing the second.

Old Body: The state your body was in before chronic pain came along.

Ownership: A perspective that defines chronic pain as a condition that you have.

Pain: An uncomfortable physical sensation, felt in one or more parts of your body, that's caused by the interaction between your mind and body and mediated by your nervous system.

Pain Avoidance: An approach to dealing with pain that directs you to run away from the pain or force it out of your life using chemicals and other treatments.

Pain Flare: An intense, and sometimes sudden, increase in your physical discomfort.

Pain Hypersensitivity: A state of increased sensitivity in your brain and nervous system that raises up your pain level.

Pain Problems: Pain-related difficulties that increase your Misery cause more pain.

Personal Comfort Approach: This invites you to take charge of your life by directing your attention towards positive thoughts, feelings, actions, and experiences that will desensitize your nervous system, reduce the influence of chronic pain, and increase your Comfort.

Positive Distractions: Activities and events that positively engage your attention.

Positive Psychology: The scientific study, and practical application, of the positive strengths that enable individuals and communities to thrive.[103]

Positive Quality: A strongly held, life affirming purpose, meaning, value, and/or ability that defines your character.

Positives: Satisfying changes and events that enhance your Comfort and sense of well-being

Recovery Time: The amount of time you spend taking a break from activities that stress your pain condition.

Re-Focusing Strategy: The practice of directing your attention towards something neutral or pleasant.

Relating Strategy: The practice of both increasing your positive connections to good people and setting limits on those who annoy you.

Relationship: A perspective that invites you to imagine that you have a relationship with pain.

Re-Thinking Strategy: The practice of moving your thinking process away from forgetfulness and negativity and towards positive well-being.

Re-Focusing Strategy: As set of Skills that direct your attention towards something neutral or pleasant.

---

[103] Adapted from the Positive Psychology Center website

Single-Focus Meditation: The practice of settling your attention on a single (or combined) focus and doing your best to keep it there (i.e., a candle flame, the breath along with a word quietly repeated in the mind).

Stressor: Something or someone that challenges, frightens, and/or pressures you.

Stress / Stress Response: Responding to a Stressor with fear, anger and other negative emotions. Brings on the fight, flight or freeze reactions.

Thought Labeling: The Mindfulness Meditation practice of noticing and mentally naming a distraction each time it comes along and then returning your attention to focus.

Toxic Talk: Messages you receive from people who criticize, manipulate, threaten, guilt trip, and generally bad mouth you. Often these words cause you to feel very uncomfortable.

Triggers: Events or situations that set off bad moods and pain flares.

Appendix G ~ Useful Books and Resources For People-in-Pain

Books about Chronic Pain, Illness, and Stress

- "Explain Pain" by David Sheridan Butler and G. Lorimer Moseley

- "A Nation in Pain: Healing Our Biggest Health Problem" by Judy Foreman

- "Pain Chronicles" by Melanie Thernstrom

- "Pain: The Science of Suffering" by Patrick Wall

- "The First Year: Irritable Bowel Syndrome," by Heather Van Vorous and David Posner

- "The First Year: Crohn's Disease and Ulcerative Colitis," by Jill Sklar

- "The First Year: H.I.V." by Brett Grodeck

- "The First Year: Fibromyalgia," by Claudia Craig Marek

- "The CFIDS/Fibromyalgia Toolkit: A Practical Self-Help Guide," by Bruce F. Campbell

- "The Complete Guide to Pain Relief," by Reader's Digest

- "Living Well with a Hidden Disability: Transcending Doubt and Shame and Reclaiming Your Life," by Stacy Taylor

- "Repetitive Strain Injury: A Computer User's Guide," by Emil Pascarelli and Deborah Quilter

- "The Pain Survival Guide," by Dennis Turk and Frits Winter

- "Numb Toes ad Aching Soles: Coping with Peripheral Neuropathy," by John A. Senneff

- "Chronic Pain Solution: Your Personal Path to Pain Relief," by James N. Dillard

- "The Truth About Chronic Pain: Patients and Professionals on How to Face it, Understand it, and Overcome it," by Arthur Rosenfeld

- "Positive Options for Reflex Sympathetic Dystrophy (RSD)," by Elena Juris (RSD is now called CRPS)

- "The War on Pain" by Scott Fishman

- "Mastering Pain: A Twelve-Step Program for Coping with Chronic Pain," by Richard Sternbach

- "The Culture of Pain," David B Morris

- "People in Pain," by Mark Zborowski (study of different social groups & how they handle pain)

- "The Relaxation and Stress reduction workbook," by Martha Davis and others

- "Conquering Your Child's Chronic Pain: A Pediatrician's Guide for Reclaiming a Normal Childhood," by Lonnie K Zeltzer

- "The Headache Sourcebook," by Joel Paulino & Ceabert J Griffith

- "Headache Free," by Roger Cady & Kathleen Farmer

- "Why Zebras Don't Get Ulcers: The Acclaimed Guide to Stress, Stress-Related Diseases, and Coping," by Robert M. Sapolsky

- "250 Tips for Making Life with Arthritis Easier," by Shelley Peterman Schwarz (for the Arthritis Foundation

- "The End of Stress as We Know It," by Bruce McEwen and Elizabeth Lasley

Books about Chronic Pain, Suffering and Spirituality

- "Turning Suffering Inside Out: A Zen Approach to Living with Physical and Emotional Pain," by Darlene Cohen

- "Chronic Pain: Finding Hope in the Midst of Suffering," by Rob Prince (a Christian perspective)

- "Making Sense of Suffering: A Jewish Approach," by Yitchok Kirzner

- "How to Be Sick: Buddhist-Inspired Guide for the Chronically Ill and Their Caregivers," by Toni Bernhard

- "Chronic Pain: Biomedical and Spiritual Approaches," by Harold Koenig

Books About Difficult Relationships and How to Deal with Them

- "When I Say No, I Feel Guilty," by Manuel J Smith

- "People Skills," by Robert Bolton

- "Perfect Phrases for Dealing with Difficult People," by Susan Benjamin

- "Nasty People: How to Stop Being Hurt by them Without Stooping to their Level," by Jay Carter

- "Dealing with People You Can't Stand," by Rick Brinkman and Rick Kirschner

- "Don't Let Your Kids Kill You," by Charles Rubin

- "Storms Can't Hurt the Sky: A Buddhist Path Through Divorce," by Gabriel Cohen

- "The Good Divorce: Keeping Your Family together When Your Marriage comes Apart," by Constance Ahrons

- "Divorce Busting: A Step-by-Step Approach to Making Your Marriage Loving Again," by Michele Weiner-Davis

Books About Hypnosis and Meditation

- "Hypnotize Yourself Out of Pain Now!" by Bruce N. Eimer

- "Hypnosis for Chronic Pain Management: Workbook," by Mark P Jensen

- "Clinical Hypnosis for Pain Control," by David R Patterson

- "Hypnosis and Hypnotherapy with Children (4th Edition)," by Daniel P. Kohen and Karen Olness

- "Hypnosis" by Ursula Markham

- "Hypnosis" by Ursula Markham

- "Essentials of Hypnosis" by Michael Yapko

- "Full Catastrophe Living: Using the Wisdom of Your Body and Mind to Face Stress, Pain, and Illness, " by Jon Kabat-Zinn

- "Altered Traits: Science Reveals How Meditation Changes Your Mind, Brain, and Body" by Daniel Goleman and Richard J Davidson

- "The Relaxation Response" by Herbert Benson

- "10% Happier" by Dan Harris

Books About Daily Activities

- "In Praise of Slowness," by Carl Honore

- "Less: Accomplishing More by Doing Less," by Marc Lesser

- "Getting Things Done," by David Allen

Books About the Mind, Brain and Nervous System

- "Train Your Mind, Change Your Brain," by Sharon Begley

- "Mindsight" – The New Science of Personal Transformation" by Daniel L Siegel

- "The Seven Sins of Memory: How the Mind Forgets and Remembers" by Daniel L. Schacter

- "The Brain that Changes Itself" by Norman Doidge

- "Your Brain on Nature" by Eva M Selhub and Allan C. Logan

- "Emotional Intelligence" by Daniel Goleman

- "Focus" by Daniel Goleman

- "Women Who Think Too Much: How to Break Free of Over-Thinking and Reclaim Your Life" by Susan Nolan-Hoeksema

Books About Positive Psychology and Happiness

- "The How of Happiness: A Scientific Approach to Getting the Life You Want," by Sonja Lyubomirsky

- "Flow," by Mihaly Csikszentmihaly

- "Positivity," by Barbara Fredrickson.

- "Thanks! – How Practicing Gratitude can Make You Happier," by Robert A. Emmons

- "Love and Survival: Eight Pathways to Intimacy and Health," by Dean Ornish

- "Learned Optimism: How to Change Your Mind and Your Life," by Martin P Seligman

- "Born to be Good," by Dacher Keltner
- "The Myths of Happiness," by Sonja Lyubomirsky

Chronic Pain & Other Educational and Support Organizations[104]

For General Public

- American Chronic Pain Association
- National Fibromyalgia and Chronic Pain Association
- American Fibromyalgia Syndrome Association
- PainEDU
- The Pain Community
- Facial Pain Association
- National Vulvodynia Association
- Pain Pathways Magazine
- Pain Connection Newsletter
- International Pain Foundation
- Campaign to End Chronic Pain in Women
- Worldwide Headache Information Center
- Cancer Pain Release
- City of Hope Pain and Palliative Care Resource Center
- Massachusetts Pain Initiative
- Pain News Network
- Milton H. Erickson Foundation Newsletter
- National Center For Complementary and Integrative Health – Chronic Pain
- American Society of Clinical Hypnosis
- Community Pain Center

---

[104] I am not promoting any particular organizations by listing them here.

For Professionals and Healthcare Providers

- International Association for the Study of Pain
- American Pain Society
- National Coalition of Chronic Pain Providers and Professionals
- Academy of Integrative Pain Management
- Practical Pain Management (journal)
- MD Magazine Pain Management
- American Academy of Pain Medicine

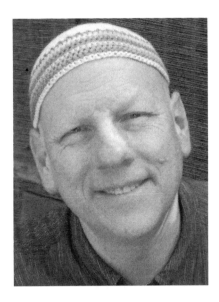

Daniel Lev, PhD is a licensed clinical psychologist who for the last twenty-five-years has taught meditation, hypnosis, and other "Comfort Skills" to help many people in chronic pain find their way to increased comfort and a better life. He has worked in many settings including Kaiser-Permanente Chronic Pain Programs, Children's Hospital Oakland, and in private medical clinics. He presently serves the people of Hawaii on the Island of Oahu through his private practice, The Comfort Clinic, and through his work in the Interdisciplinary Pain Program of Premier Medical Group-Hawaii. You can contact him through ComfortClinic.org.

Made in the USA
San Bernardino, CA
28 April 2018